COLLECT
WHAT YOU
PRODUCE!

COLLECT
WHAT YOU
PRODUCE!

CATHY JAMESON, M.A.

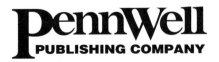

PUBLISHING COMPANY

DENTAL ECONOMICS

PennWell Publishing Company
Tulsa, Oklahoma

Also by Cathy Jameson, M.A.
Great Communication = Great Production
PennWell Books ISBN 087814-427-7
Also Available on Audiotape

Cover photography by John Trammel Photography, Oklahoma City, OK.

Copyright 1996 by
PennWell Publishing Company
1421 South Sheridan Road/P.O. Box 1260
Tulsa, OK 74101-1260

Jameson, Cathy.
    Collect What You Produce! / by Cathy Jameson.
       p.   cm.
    Includes index.
    ISBN 0-87814-588-5
    1. Dental fees. 2. Collecting of accounts. I. Title.
    [DNLM: 1. Practice Management, Dental—economics.   2. Economics, Dental.   3. Financial
Management. WU 77 J31c 1996]
RK58.J35 1996
617.6′0068′1—dc20
DNLM/DLC
for Library of Congress   96-15336
                                                                CIP

Printed in the United States of America
1 2 3 4 5 00 99 98 97 96

DEDICATION

To the many mentors, teachers, and friends who have guided, directed, coached, and taught me along my path of learning. Thanks for the information, the knowledge, the wisdom, and the encouragement.

To John, my husband, best friend, soulmate, companion, sounding board, and my favorite dentist!

Contents

Introduction

Professional success depends on learning business skills and people skills. Financial arrangements are business skills that are focused on taking care of people's financial issues. Making proper financial arrangements with the patient before treatment is rendered serves both the patient and the dentist. Carefully and caringly informing patients about their financial responsibilities offsets many potential problems and misunderstandings. In addition, cost is one of—if not the greatest—barrier to treatment acceptance. People may want or need the dental care that you are recommending but feel they cannot afford it. Therefore, finding solutions to the financial issues of your patients is critical if your practice is to thrive. You want and need to provide the treatment. You need to be paid for that treatment. And, you need to have options available that will work for the vast majority of your patients. Thus, this book. It is my intention to give you solid advice, thorough instruction, and necessary armamentarium to make and carry out successful financial arrangements with your patients.

A successful business is built upon carefully established and effectively administered systems. A dental practice is a business and, therefore, is dependent upon the quality of its systems. The financial aspect of your practice is a system—or actually, a sequence of systems. The goal of these systems is to accomplish the following:

- Make the financing of your patient's dental care comfortable so that the vast majority of patients will be able to "go ahead" with necessary and desired treatment.

- "Collect what you produce" to insure a healthy cash flow in your practice.

- Increase patient flow and gain a higher case acceptance.

- Reduce the amount of time your team members spend on statements and collection so that they can spend time on practice building and patient service.

- Reduce or eliminate private pay accounts receivable. Make sure that your accounts receivable is no more than 1 to 1½ times your average monthly production. (This will be mostly outstanding insurance.)

There are approximately 20 different systems that make up a dental practice. The financing system seems to present more challenges for the practice and for the members of the team than any of the other systems. Why? There are several reasons.

1. No clear definition of policy is in place and the people administering the practice have no guidelines to follow.

2. Sometimes dental team members are uncomfortable with their own fees—or with discussion of fees; therefore, patients become uncomfortable.

3. Excellent training in the area of financing is not provided for the team members, and the people who are expected to carry out financial responsibilities do so without the necessary expertise.

4. Some dentists feel that they should "give away" their services.

5. Team members get "gun shy" when patients protest about fees and think that they must compromise fees or become extremely lenient in financial arrangements so that people will accept treatment recommendations.

6. Communication skills that define a patient's financial concerns and clarify arrangements have not been taught.

WHY THIS BOOK?

As a management consultant, I have rarely gone into a practice where a clear and effective financial system is in place. Thus, financial stress becomes a challenge for the practice and for the practitioner. My work at the Master's and Doctoral level has been focused on "Controlling Stress in the Dental Environment".

WHY?

My dentist husband, Dr. John Jameson, and I have experienced just about every kind of problem and every kind of stress known to dental man or woman. Stress can be good. That's what gets you up every morning. Positive stress gives you the ambition to study and become better at what you do. However, when stress becomes negative—when it leads to mental, psychological, and physical discomfort and illness—it becomes distress. That's what I want to help you avoid—distress. Having lived through most dental trials and tribulations, I have become committed to helping our dental colleagues avoid or overcome situations that lead to distress.

Can a book on financing serve this purpose? Yes. John and I have known all stresses, but we both feel that nothing has been more difficult than financial stress. Financial stress takes away

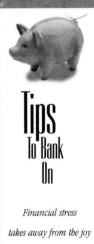

Tips To Bank On

Financial stress takes away from the joy of dentistry

from the joy of dentistry, it can hinder associations with patients, and it can have a negative effect on personal relationships—particularly marriages!

GOALS

Over the last decade I have spent much time studying financing in order to deal with negative factors that impact a practice's financial security. My goal in writing this book is to give you the armamentarium to establish a quality financial system that will make the financing of your services comfortable for your patients and for you. I plan to give you not only the instruction necessary to develop this system, but also the management tools and the communication skills to gain success in this area of your practice.

The following goals will be pursued:

- Establish a clear financial policy that will produce a **win-win** situation for the patients and the practice.

- Teach the communication skills necessary to positively present the financial options.

- Establish a protocol for identifying and overcoming the objections that are related to the fee for dental services.

- Motivate you to get involved with a healthcare financing program and then have the ability to market and build the practice by using the program.

- Give you the skills necessary to become insurance aware but not insurance driven.

- Get control of your collection system so that you "collect what you produce."

- Help you become comfortable with the financial aspect of your practice so that all members of the team feel good about the system and are confident with the proper administration of that system.

YOU ARE WORTH IT!

As healthcare providers, you are offering a significant service to your patients—a service that establishes health and beauty. What you do for patients enhances their life, their health, and their self esteem. When patients perceive the quality of care they are receiving in your practice and when they see their dental care as a significant benefit, they will be more than happy to pay for the services. You will have fewer complaints about money and you will not have people asking you to compromise your treatment plans or your fees.

It is impossible to write a book about financing or to discuss this "system" in a consultation or lecture without establishing the point that when patients perceive quality and benefit of care, they will feel that the exchange of value—money for service—is equitable. Didn't Dr. Pankey teach us that some time ago? It remains true, now and always.

STEP ONE: ATTITUDE

If I could ask you for one thing as you begin reading this book and initiating your study and implementation of the system, it would be this: Please open your mind.

> "A mind is like a parachute, it only works when it is open."
>
> — KEVIN MURPHY
> *EFFECTIVE LISTENING*

This quotation says it all, doesn't it! I may reinforce and repeat things that you already know and are doing. If so, pat

Tips To Bank On

When patients perceive the quality of care they are receiving in your practice and when they see their dental care as a significant benefit, they will be more than happy to pay for the services.

yourself on the back and keep on doing those things. Don't just think, "Oh, we already do that. We don't need to study that". Not so. Repetition is the key to learning. If I talk about things that you are already doing, be proud. But, also look for little things that you can do to refine what you are already doing. Be a committed student. Always be in the business of self improvement.

On the other hand, I may ask you to step out of your comfort zone. I will introduce you to things that you may not have heard before. I will be teaching you some communication skills that you have not used before. Know that these communication skills are "tried and true". Study the new skills. Practice with commitment. Constantly refine and improve your skills.

Most of all, just like anything, you will get out of the book exactly what you put into it. Know that if you use a part of the skills, you will get partial success. If you implement all of the skills, you will gain incredible success.

Dental professionals would never implement a *portion* of a clinical system and expect success. If you did only a part of a crown procedure, you would not expect for the procedure to end in success. You do the whole thing—step by step—consistently. Not once, but every time. Thus, the law of averages is in your favor and you gain success most every time you do a crown.

However, people do not transfer that same commitment to their management systems. They think they can take one idea out of a presentation or a book and that they will gain great success. Not so! A management system—such as financing—takes the same commitment to consistency; consistency in administration of the system, all of it, every time. Then, the law of averages takes your side, and success will be yours.

Read. Study. Have staff meetings about each chapter. Use this book as a textbook on financing. It is just that. Make a commitment to implement all the strategies. The results will be the following:

- increased cash flow,

- less time and money spent on collections, thus reducing overhead,

- greater treatment acceptance, therefore higher productivity,

- reduced stress, and

- fun.

I hope that the study of this material and the implementation of the system will increase the joy that you receive in the practice of dentistry. Enjoy!

Establishing the Financial System in Your Practice

> "Everyone can take part in a team.
> The aim of a team is to improve the input and
> the output of any stage. A team may well be
> composed of people from different staff areas.
> A team has a customer."
>
> —W. EDWARD DEMING
> OUT OF THE CRISIS

In order for the financial system of your practice to be clear and comfortable, a written policy needs to be established and put into place. As I consult across the country and throughout the world, I rarely go into a practice where a written financial policy is in place. Most practices figure out how they are going to handle the financial aspect of a patient's treatment as they go. The financial system in the practice is a "guess and by golly" system that changes as moods change!

Therefore, establishing a "firm yet flexible" system of financial options—or establishing a financial policy—is one of the first

Tips
To Bank
On

The oral cavity is an

intimate zone of a

person's body.

So is the pocketbook.

and most critical steps in developing a well managed dental practice. No one wins when there is a lack of clarity in this sensitive area, financing. The oral cavity is an intimate zone of a person's body. So is the pocketbook. That's why it is so important that a person's financial responsibility be clearly defined and mutually agreed upon.

Without a set policy, this would be next to impossible. Trying to figure out what you are going to do with a patient's financial responsibility without any guidelines leads to confusion. A confused person cannot make a decision. Therefore, without clarity in the area of financing you run the risk of a patient not accepting treatment, putting treatment off, or having to "think about it". Neither you nor the patient wins. You do not get to provide the treatment and the patient does not receive the necessary or desired care.

ESTABLISHMENT OF A FINANCIAL SYSTEM

Seven steps need to be taken to establish and implement a financial system.

1. **Set and write the policy.** A written financial policy is essential. Making arbitrary, random decisions about *who's* going to pay and *how* they will pay will lead to financial chaos for your practice. Loss of control of accounts receivable can result. Problems and misunderstandings from patients in regard to their financial responsibility can arise.

   Historically, many dentists have feared setting a firm financial policy because they thought that patients would leave the practice if they weren't "lenient" with the financial aspect of treatment. A good financial policy will allow for desired flexibility but also will provide necessary firmness for practice solidity.

2. **Decide, as a team, what financial options you are going to make available.** "If a person is allowed to be a part of a decision-making process, that person will be

more likely to *buy into* the decision". Abiding by this proven management principle, you will see that if the entire team understands the financial options and decides—together—which options are applicable and appropriate to your practice, they will support the policy. They will be confident that the policy serves both the practice and the patients and will not hesitate to discuss the policy with patients.

If a team member questions the financial policy, that lack of confidence will come through *loud and clear* to patients. *Their* insecurity will lead to *patient* insecurity.

3. **Financial arrangements *must* be made before any treatment is provided.** Patients have made it clear that they don't like "not knowing how much the treatment will cost before it's done". We *must* listen to our consumers/patients and respond positively to what they are requesting. They are saying "Let me know, in advance, what my financial responsibility will be". Mutual respect will result.

Establishing clarity in regard to a patient's financial responsibility before treatment is rendered will reduce post treatment misunderstandings and quarrels about the fee for the service and about payment responsibilities. Most of the time when a patient leaves the practice unhappy, the cause is a misunderstanding about money.

Some dental professionals think that if they talk about the financial responsibility before treatment is rendered, the patient will think that all they care about is money. Not so! Listen carefully. People say, according to the American Dental Association, that the thing they like least about dental appointments is not knowing how much a procedure will cost before it is performed. Therefore, spending quality time with a patient explaining the fee for the service, discussing the options available for payment, and coming to terms with an agreed upon payment arrangement is *exactly* what the patients are asking you to do. They will not resent this. They will appreciate this.

4. **Designate a specific person on the team to administer financial arrangements.** Establish who, when, where, and how this person will make the financial arrangements.

This person, probably the business administrator or the treatment coordinator, will review the treatment plan that the doctor has discussed, define the fees, analyze expected insurance, (if applicable), and work with a patient to determine the financial option that is acceptable. A financial agreement would be *written* so that neither party would *forget* or become *confused* about the agreement.

The dentist may quote the fee, but it is usually more effective for a business administrator to make the financial arrangements. A qualified business administrator can give necessary third party reinforcement to the dentist's recommendations, making sure that there are no clinical questions that have been left unanswered. Patients may be more comfortable discussing financial concerns with the administrator rather than the dentist. In addition, the person who has been given the responsibility of handling the financial aspect of the practice will be less likely to make alterations to the financial policy.

Critical Point: If a person is given the responsibility to implement and carry out a financial policy, then she must have the support of the dentist and the entire team. Nothing is more debilitating, embarrassing, and frustrating than to be very clear and very good at making a financial arrangement only to be undermined by the dentist or other team members. This is why the entire team needs to decide what financial options will be made available. This will give everyone the confidence that the arrangement will be good for the patient and for the practice. This support if absolutely necessary if this is going to work.

With any system, program, or policy you need to be consistent in the administration of the system. Nevertheless, you also need to know when to *flex*. Determine situations that warrant *flexing*. However, do not make flexing the rule, make it the exception.

Tips To Bank On

CRITICAL POINT:

If a person is given the responsibility to implement and carry out a financial policy, then she must have the support of the dentist and the entire team.

Special Note: In our own practice, our business administrator joins the dentist and the patient for the consultation appointment. The dentist asks the patient for permission. He says, "Ms. Jones, I've asked Jan, my business administrator, to join us today for our consultation. Jan handles the financial arrangements for our patients and she schedules the appointments. Therefore, I feel it is important for her to hear the recommendations that I'm making for you. Are you comfortable with that?" (No one has ever said "No".)

The dentist presents his recommendations, answers treatment questions, asks for the commitment to go ahead with treatment, then—when there are no other questions except financing—he excuses himself. The business administrator/treatment coordinator takes over. She reconfirms the treatment, answers any clinical questions where confusion may exist, defines the total investment, and the financial options available for payment. Together, she and the patient clarify all financial responsibilities. She writes this down on our written financial agreement. Then, she schedules the first appointment.

5. **Do *your* best to create a time and a place for private consultation—both clinical and financial.** As I said earlier, the oral cavity is an intimate zone of the body. So is the pocketbook! To discuss treatment recommendations or financing in public is uncomfortable and awkward. This could become a hindrance to a person accepting and going ahead with treatment.

   Find the place! Create the appropriate environment! It doesn't have to be fancy. It just has to *work!* Schedule the time for this consultation. This financial consultation is as critical as any phase of your treatment!

6. **Study communication skills relative to establishing a financial arrangement and handling objections.** The bottom line to your success in any of the systems in your practice is the way you communicate. Whether you are answering the telephone, presenting the treatment plan, scheduling appointments or determining the financial arrangement, the way you communicate will make all the difference in the world.

Tips
To Bank
On

See Special Note:

Tips
To Bank
On

The bottom line to your success in any of the systems in your practice is the way you communicate.

Paul Harvey says, "It's not what you say, it's how you say it." Don't you agree? You can present the financial options in one way and get a negative reaction from the patient, but present it in another way and establish an open, accepting, negotiating relationship. Clear communication is necessary if a mutually respectful relationship is to evolve and treatment acceptance is to result.

7. **Analyze your fees at least every six months.** Notice that I didn't say raise your fees every six months, but I did say analyze your fees every six months. If the cost of a procedure has increased due to increased cost of product, increased lab fees, or increased overhead, then you must increase the fee for that procedure. You must be willing and able to pass your increased costs of operation on to your consumers, the patients, or otherwise, you may become productive without becoming profitable.

WORKABLE FINANCIAL OPTIONS

The following is a financial policy and a series of financial options that will work for any practice, large or small, new or established, urban or rural. The options that I am recommending do, indeed, offer flexibility as well as firmness. These options will meet the needs of most of your patients. In addition, consistently following this program will get you out of the banking business and will let you concentrate on what you do best, practice dentistry.

Other benefits of this policy are as follows:

- lower cost of operation in the area of financial management,

- less time spent on statements and collection by your team members,

- greater cash flow,

- more people accepting more treatment,

- enhanced scheduling.

Patients will be able to receive more treatment per appointment and will be required to come to the office for fewer visits. You will be able to see fewer patients per day doing more dentistry per patient and see each patient for fewer visits. Everyone wins and your costs of operation are reduced significantly.

Option #1. A 5% Accounting Reduction for Payment in Full—Before Treatment is Rendered. For those patients who have healthy savings or checking accounts, this option gives them an incentive to pay in advance. Anyone who has ever been responsible for scheduling will also agree that if patients pay for the treatment in advance, they will show up for those appointments! How do you present this option?

> **Business Administrator:** "Mrs. Smith, would you be interested in having your fee reduced?

> **Mrs. Smith:** "Of course. How do I do that?"

> **Business Administrator:** "If you pay for your services before the dentist provides the treatment, we will reduce your fee by 5%. If we are not responsible for the bookkeeping, that saves us time and money. We pass those savings on to you. Would this be of interest to you?"

Many patients take advantage of this option. You are *dollars ahead* to offer this reduction versus carrying any accounts on your own books.

Option #2. Payment by the Appointment. In order to offer this financial option, the business administrator must have a complete treatment plan from the clinical team. It would be impossible to inform a person of his/her financial responsibility per appointment if you are not sure what kind of treatment is going to be provided at the next appointment.

The treatment plan must provide complete information. Just saying that you are going to do some "fillings" doesn't work. How many teeth? How many surfaces? What type of material?

Amalgam or composite? All of these details are necessary before proper financial discussions can take place.

If you are discussing a full treatment plan that will involve several appointments, and if the person needs to spread his/her payments out over the course of the treatment, do so in the following manner: (1) determine the total fee, (2) divide the fee equally into the number of appointments, (3) determine a specific series of dates that payments will be expected during the course of the treatment, (4) make sure that full payment is accomplished by the end of the treatment.

If you figure the payment due at each particular appointment, you run the risk of the patient falling out of treatment. They may complete only a part of the treatment and then decide they don't want to spend any more money. By dividing the fee into equal payments spread over the course of treatment, you reduce that possibility.

Option #3. Insurance on Assignment. A recent ADA survey asked people across the entire country the following question, "If you needed to make a one-time dental purchase of $500, could you?" 77% of the people who responded said, "No!"

Understanding this critical fact, I usually recommend taking insurance on assignment. If you are in a high socioeconomic area and if your patients can afford to pay for their care and wait for the insurance company to reimburse them directly, then by all means, do just that! That's the best!

However, for the vast majority of practices, not accepting assignment would eliminate a great many patients and a great deal of dentistry.

Insurance management is not easy. You must have an effective, efficient system in place. (We will discuss a method of managing your insurance in a later chapter.) The financial reward and the service to your patients makes the effort worthwhile.

With this knowledge from your consumers, let's evaluate a hypothetical situation: Ms. Jones comes to the office and the dentist diagnoses the need for $1000 worth of dentistry. You say "Ms. Jones, we need for you to pay for the treatment today in full. We will give you the necessary paperwork and you can file your own insurance. Then your insurance company will reimburse you."

Again, if your patients can afford to do this, great! It's the best way. However, many patients in the United States today would not receive the treatment if this was the only option available. Most patients, if asked to take care of the $1000 charge and wait for their insurance company to reimburse them would say,"I can't afford to do this right now. I'll call you." *There* are the three most dangerous words in dentistry—"I'll call you". Why? Because, most of the time they won't.

Therefore, handling insurance is a critical system within the practice and deserves respect and attention. But I do recommend—in most practices—that you accept dental insurance.

Option #4. Mastercard/VISA/Discover/American Express.

These wonderful financing vehicles have not, historically, been used extensively to finance dentistry. In fact, only a small percentage of the dentistry in the U.S. is financed with bank cards.

However, this trend is on an upward swing. The major bank cards are making significant efforts to capture a larger segment of the healthcare market. They are informing the public that using a bank card for the financing of dental/medical care makes good sense. These wonderful companies can afford to market to the consumer in a large way. Every dental office will be a benefactor of their brilliant marketing efforts.

Dr. Charles Blair, Charlotte, NC asked the readers of his financial management newsletter the following questions, "Would you use a bank card to finance your dental care?" Approximately 75% of the respondents said "Yes." However, only 6% of the dentistry in the United States is being financed on a bank card presently. So, Dr. Blair asked the next question, "Most of you say that you would use a bank card to finance your dental care, but only 6% of you are doing so. Why?" The answers were: (1) "My dentist doesn't accept bank cards." and (2) "I don't know if my dentist accepts bank cards."

In a recent interview, VISA asked me, "Cathy, do you recommend that dentists market the use of a bank card to their patients?" I answered without hesitation, "Yes!" Informing your own patient family—and the people within your drawing area—of the fact the bank cards are accepted and encouraged in your practice can make the difference in whether a family comes to you or not and in whether a person accepts treatment recommendations or not.

You must *ask* for these cards. Don't just hang up a sign and think people will respond. You have to mention and *encourage* the use of this option. In your patient education newsletters, special mailings, telephone ads, newspaper announcements, on your statements, and during your financial consultations, ask people to use this option. Encourage people. Inform them of the benefits of financing with a bank card.

Call VISA—toll free—1-800-VISA-311 and ask for their "Healthcare Marketing Packet". Included in this packet are brochures about VISA for your patients, pre-authorization forms, and stickers to be placed on your statements. Contact the other bank card programs and ask for available materials to market their bank card to your patients.

Market the option of a bankcard to your patients. Do not be one of those dentists who doesn't accept VISA, Mastercard, and Discover. Do not be one of those dentists who has not informed his/her patients—on a regular basis—about the advantages of using a bank card for the financing of dental care.

Bank cards are *very* desirable options. Don't worry about the service charge. Running your own credit business is financially devastating and inadequate at best.

Option #5. Post-Dated Checks or Three Pre-Signed Bank Card Vouchers, or Pre-Authorization for Payments on a Bank Card.

According to leaders in the collection industry, 95-98% of all post-dated checks clear the bank. If a patient wants to make two or three equal payments, the option of post-dated checks or pre-signed bank card vouchers is acceptable and encouraged. Check with your own state to see if there are any specifics relative to your state. However, in most states this is a perfectly legal method of scheduling payments. The verbal skills of presenting this option are critical:

> **Ms. Jones:** "Can I just pay you for this crown over a few months?"

Tips To Bank On

Call VISA—toll free—

1-800-VISA-311

and ask for their

"Healthcare Marketing

Packet".

Business Administrator: "Yes, Ms. Jones, we can make that possible. The way we handle that type of payment schedule is three equal payments with post-dated checks. The first one-third is due at the time of the service. The next one-third is due 30 days after that. The final one-third is due 30 days after that. Or, if you prefer, we could accept three pre-signed vouchers from your bank card. Which would you prefer?"

Consider using bank card pre-authorization forms! (See Fig. 1–1)   If you make an arrangement with a patient to use a

---

You may create your own Pre-Authorized Health Care Form or reproduce this one onto your letterhead

Pre-Authorized Health Care Form

I authorize _____

_____
(name of health care provider)

to keep my signature on file and to charge my Visa® account for:

☐ Balance of charges not paid by insurance within 90 days and not to exceed $ _____ for:
    ☐ this visit only
    ☐ all visits this year

☐ Recurring charges (ongoing treatments) of $ _____

every _____
    (frequency)

from _____ to _____
    (date)   (date)

I assign my insurand benefits to the provider listed above. I understand that this form is valid for one year unless I cancel the authorization through written notice to the health provider.

Patient Name: _____

Cardholder Name: _____

Cardholder Address: _____

City: _____

State: _____ Zip: _____

Account Number: _____

Expiration Date: _____

Cardholder Signature: _____

Date: _____

Figure 1–1

bank card, you can have him/her fill out one of the bank card pre-authorization forms. You would need to make a note in your tickler file as to when the vouchers are to be mailed to the bank card company. Then, simply complete the charge slip, send a copy to the bank card company or use an automatic "swipe" machine, and then send a copy of the voucher to the patient. Last, but not least, adjust your bank deposit in the positive. No statements. No collection efforts. Good for you. Good for the patient.

Option #6. For Any Long Term or Extended Payments, a Healthcare Financing Program. These programs have become a tremendous asset to the dental industry by providing convenient financing for comprehensive—or immediate—care.

Use of these programs gets you, the dentist, out of the banking business while still allowing patients the opportunity to spread the payment of treatment out over several months. Monthly payments are small and fit comfortably into the family budget.

Most people need some financial assistance if they are to receive the treatment that is recommended to them. Remember the study performed by the American Dental Association. "If you needed to make a one time dental purchase of $500, could you?" Seventy-seven percent of the American population said "no", that they could not afford a one time dental purchase of $500. (77% of Americans) You and I both know that $500 can't even buy a crown, let alone a root canal, post and core, and a crown!

Most people live on budgets and are not as concerned about how much the total investment will be as they are about how they can pay for it, or if they can make payments, or how much they will pay per month.

That is why you must offer a payment option that answers the financial needs of the people, helps them to receive quality care, and helps the practice to be financially solid. The answer is to offer a healthcare financing program to those folks who need financial assistance to access the necessary or desired care.

Example: A person comes into your office with some discomfort. You recommend endodontic therapy followed by a crown. We know that 77% of the people probably cannot afford that kind of necessary treatment unless their insurance company is going to pay the vast majority of it or they have some method of "paying it out". They aren't saying "I don't want this treatment." They are asking for help—financial help. They are saying, "Help me find a solution to my problem—my money problem". If you have done a good job of presenting the dentistry, and they want the treatment, they may just need a way to pay for it.

However, if you become the bank and if you loan the patient the money for the treatment, you add a costly dimension to your practice—you open a banking business within the practice and most dental professionals are not financial, business, or banking experts. They are dental professionals and are better off doing what they know best—dentistry—and turning the financing over to professionals in *that* field.

How many patients come to the business office and say, "I really want this treatment. I know I need this. Can I pay it out or can I make payments to you"? The minute the patient says, "Doctor, can I pay this out?" and you say, "Yes", then you become a lending institution and you add to the overhead of your practice—significantly. Ultimately, it is not financially wise for you to run a banking business within your practice. However, most people need long term financing to be able to receive any extensive treatment. Thus, for any long-term or extended payment, offer a healthcare financing program. A healthcare financing system does the following:

1. Provides financial assistance for healthcare only. It is not a service that is in competition with other bank cards. It is not in competition with food, entertainment, clothes, or vacations, etc. This type of program allows families and individuals to establish a line of credit for healthcare.

2. People can receive needed or desired care, the best available, but make small monthly payments and spread those payments out over a comfortable length of time, dependent upon how much they can afford to pay per month. Thus, the total investment does not become such

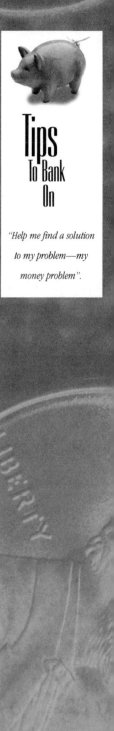

Tips To Bank On

"Help me find a solution to my problem—my money problem".

an enormous barrier. Accessing a comfortable monthly investment becomes the solvable challenge.

3. People do not have to go to a location outside of the office to apply for this line of credit. They apply right there in your office. The dentist pays all necessary enrollment fees and there is no annual fee.

4. If a patient has dental insurance but cannot afford the balance after insurance, the patient can place the balance on his/her financing program. He/she can use the healthcare financing program in conjunction with their dental insurance. This will let them better use the insurance benefits they have already paid for.

5. These financing programs also have pre-authorizations so that patients can give you permission to place any balance after insurance pays or for you to place regular monthly payments on their line of credit. Once a person gets involved with one of these financing programs, be sure to get a signed pre-authorization form in his/her chart to use in either one of these situations.

WHAT IF THE PATIENT DOESN'T GET ACCEPTED?

There are different types of healthcare financing programs. (See Appendix A for a partial listing of available companies) Most of the programs are non-recourse, which means that if the patient doesn't pay, you are not responsible for the account. One of the major differences in the programs is the acceptance rate—how many people are going to be approved for a line of credit.

It can become very discouraging to an office to see the benefit of such a financial service, recommend the service, get people to fill out the applications, only to have patients denied, time and time again. These offices get so discouraged with the programs that they are afraid to present this option. And, on the other hand, the patients are placed in an embarrassing situation where the dental team now knows that they cannot receive a line of credit.

The key to the success of your program is to study the variances of the programs carefully. Contact the companies listed in the Appendix A. Ask each company about their approval rate in your area. Call other offices in your area who are using the program and find out what their acceptance rate has been. Then, select a program that will meet your needs and the needs of your patients—one that has a high acceptance rate in your area.

Not every patient will get accepted, no matter how high the acceptance rate of the company. The fact that the company will be doing a very careful credit rating and screening of the patient will help you to make better business decisions about financing your dentistry. If a patient is *not* granted a line of credit with your program, ask yourself this question,"Do we want to make a loan to this patient if the professional financial people are unwilling to do so?" Probably not. Rather, you may need to back off the treatment plan just a bit and do a tooth at a time—based on the patient's ability to pay as they go—or "payment by the appointment".

Another way to deal with the patient who is not granted a line of credit is to do "lay away dentistry". This means that the patient makes monthly payments to you. You place these payments in an account as a growing "credit". Then, when he/she has the money saved, you can proceed with the dentistry. We have many patients who participate in this program and are happy to receive the care without having financial stress added to their lives.

Many times we do "just because" dentistry. John provides care for a person "just because". He would rather provide free care as a chosen "love gift" instead of making an unrealistic financial arrangement with a person only to be disappointed or to be placed in a costly situation of having to try to collect an uncollectable account.

In certain situations, we refer patients to the dental school for care by the students. These students will, of course, provide excellent care. This is an excellent service to both the indigent family and to the students.

WHAT IF AN EMERGENCY NEEDS FINANCIAL ASSISTANCE?

If a person comes to your practice in an emergency situation, follow these protocols:

- Determine, on the phone, if the patient is an emergency. Use a patient communication slip to gather necessary information. Then, if the patient does have an emergency situation, see the person that day. (Fig. 1–2)

- On the telephone, let the patient know that he/she will be expected to pay the fee for the emergency visit at the time of the service. Then, let him/her know that if the dentist needs to provide treatment, there will be a financial discussion before any treatment is rendered and that the patient will not be put in a position for any financial surprises.

- If the person indicates a concern about finances, inform him/her of your financial options. If he/she is uncomfortable with cash payments and he/she does not have a bank card, introduce him/her to your healthcare financing program. Ask the patient to come in earlier than the scheduled time to complete an application. Then, while the patient is waiting to be seated, or certainly before the dentist renders any treatment beyond the emergency care, you will know whether or not he/she has been extended a line of credit and, if so, for how much.

  This is valuable information. You do not know this person. You do not need to make your own loan to him/her. However, you do want to provide the necessary care. By establishing a line of credit for the person with your financing company, both of these needs are fulfilled.

- If the patient comes in for the emergency visit and the dentist diagnoses necessary treatment and wants to go ahead with that treatment while the patient is there, two things must be in place:

1. You must have the time to render that treatment without that having a negative affect on your regularly scheduled patients. If you do not have

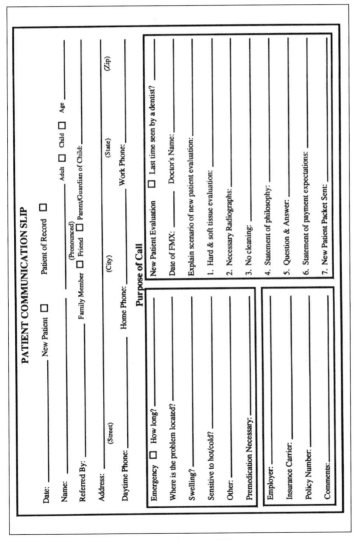

Figure 1–2 Patient Communication Slip

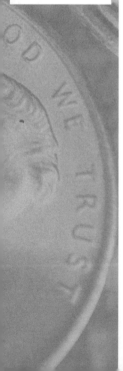

the time, diagnose, prescribe treatment, get the patient comfortable, and reschedule him/her for the necessary length of time. A trauma case would be an exception. Otherwise, you need to respect the time of your regularly scheduled patients. Palliative treatment only!

2. Inform the patient of the financial responsibility before treatment is rendered. Patients *want* to know what is expected of them financially before the fact. In addition, you run the risk of acquiring a bad debt if you do not handle the financial aspect of an emergency visit as carefully as you handle the clinical aspects.

While a patient is in the chair and you diagnose necessary treatment, if there is time to do that treatment, have the business administrator step back to the clinical area to discuss the fee and the options for payment. If the patient needs financial assistance, get an application for your financial program, help him/her to complete the application, then modem, fax, or call the information to your particular company. You will know in a matter of minutes whether or not the patient has been extended that line of credit and for how much. Then, let the dentist know that he/she can go ahead with the treatment or that he/she needs to consider some other alternative.

This procedure only takes a few minutes and can make a big difference in your financial security. If you analyze your accounts receivable carefully, you may find that a healthy portion of those accounts may be emergency patients who never had a financial arrangement made and who never paid.

You are there to work with the patient. It's OK for them to be asked to work with you.

How Do You Get Started?

There are many excellent programs on the market today. Gather the information on the programs listed in the Appendix and any others that you may know. Write or call the companies for a packet of material. Study that information. Add this service to your practice. Your challenge is to do enough research to find out which program will fit your practice, your geographic area, and your socio-economic situation.

There is a service fee for these programs. After you read the next chapter you will see that the service fee is miniscule compared to how much it costs for you to carry accounts on your own books. There are significant differences in the service fee that each company charges the dentist. The differences are related to the amount of risk, or the number of patients that a company is willing and able to approve for credit. The higher the acceptance rate, the higher the service fee. You must determine how much of your practice population needs long term financing in order to receive the dental care and how much you are willing to invest to make that happen.

You will be making an investment in the service fee. However, in the next chapter I will prove to you, beyond a shadow of a doubt, that the service fee will be less than it is costing you right now to be running a banking business in your own practice.

IN ADDITION

Certainly, if you are recommending and presenting a large treatment plan to a patient and he/she needs financial assistance, do not forget to recommend that he/she go to a banker to apply for a loan. If the patient pays you in full before treatment begins, go ahead and offer the 5% *accounting reduction.* This will help a patient with the ensuing interest.

There are also major financing programs throughout the country that are making six-month or one year loans to patients for a specific treatment plan. These loans are interest free to the patient. The dental office pays a service fee. The patient receives the loan and the treatment—then pays the loan back with equal monthly payments—again, interest free. This type of program in your practice is a must.

Option #7.   Electronic Funds Transfer. Companies are emerging throughout the country that assist you in accessing regular withdrawals from a patient's checking or savings account.   These programs put a portion of the costs of carrying accounts into the hands of professionals.   In addition, the patients will be more likely to cover these withdrawals from a professional service than they would be inclined to send you a check following the receipt of a statement from your office.

The patient completes the necessary paperwork. Together you agree upon the date of the withdrawal as well as the designated amount. The paperwork is given to the appropriate bank. Then, withdrawals begin.

People are not unfamiliar with this type of payment option. Many home mortgage, car, and savings plan programs are a withdrawal system. Certainly, specific criteria must be in place. But, for the most part everyone has a checking account and can place a wihdrawal program into effect. If a withdrawal does not clear, the bank will put it through again. Any charges will be filed against the patient.

Another type of bank account withdrawal program establishes a system of pre-authorized checking (PAC). Patients choose the date of payment, the amount of payment, and the appropriate checking account to be accessed.   Checks are produced. The dental practice holds the pre-authorized checks in the office until the designated date of deposit. Then the check is sent in. If an emergency does arise, a patient can call the office and ask that the check deposit be delayed for a specific period of time.

While these programs do not put the money into your hands at the beginning of treatment, like the healthcare financing programs, they do eliminate the sending of statements and need for collections. You do not wait for payments, operating costs are reduced, case acceptance will increase because of the elimination of the cost barrier, and your team can focus on practice building. Check into these programs.

As You Begin to Make This Change

It will be a much easier to inform your new patients of your financial options than it will be to reeducate your existing patient family. In the following chapters I review several ways to introduce your existing patient population of the financial options—both in writing and in your verbal skills.

However, you may want to inform your existing patient family of the changes in a special mailing before those changes begin. I would recommend that you do this. In a special letter, introduce your patient family to the new financial options, concentrating on how these options will benefit them as well as the practice. (Fig. 1–3) Mail this letter 30 days before you make

---

Dear Patient Friends,

Containing the costs of healthcare has been a subject of great interest to all of us over the last few years. We, too, are interested in containing costs so that you and your family can receive quality, individualized care.

Experts in the field of management have helped us learn new and better ways to serve our patients while remaining constant in our commitment to excellent dental care. After a thorough analysis of our practice, experts made many recommendations. One of those recommendations was to offer a series of financial options to our patients so that the financing of their dental care would be comfortable. Also we learned that offering these financial options will help us to maintain reasonable fees.

Our costs of operation are soaring. But, we do not want to lower our standards of care and we do not want to go sky high with our fees. Therefore, we are implementing the following financial policy starting on January 1, 1996. This policy will offer numerous ways for you to handle the financial responsibility of your dental care.

Figure 1–3

We believe that this policy will prove to be a service to you and to your family.

1. A 5% reduction in your fee if you pay for services in advance of treatment.

2. Payment by the appointment. (This option lets you spread out the payments according to your treatment plan.)

3. Mastercard, Visa, Discover, American Express. (This option will let you know how much your monthly payments will be so that you can budget your payments comfortably.)

4. Insurance on assignment. (We will file your insurance as a service to you and will do our very best to maximize your benefits. We accept assignment of benefits to lower your immediate 'out of pocket' expenditures. We ask that you take care of your estimated portion of payment at the time of the service. We will file your insurance at the same time.)

5. 12-month interest free financing through our financing partner, XYZ Financial Company

6. For any long term or extended payments we offer ABC. (ABC is a financing program for dentistry that lets you make small monthly payments spreading those payments out over a desired period of time.)

These financial options will meet the needs of most families in our practice. We want to be flexible in changing times. We have listened to your concerns and have made great efforts to respond to those concerns. We will do our very best to work out a financial solution to your particular situation. We are here to help you.

Yours for Better Dental Health,

Figure 1–3 (continued)

the changes in policy. This will help your business administrators make a smooth transition. Then, as patients are flowing through the practice introduce them to the options (see verbal skill scripts in chapter 3).

SUMMARY

Step one in gaining control of the financial "system" in your practice is to establish a written financial policy—one that offers flexibility for your patient's needs and convenience, and one that offers firmness for the financial security of your practice. The above recommended financial policy meets the needs of the vast majority of people. People who have healthy savings and checking accounts are offered an incentive to pay in advance. People who want to take care of their payments as treatment proceeds are offered that option. Those who have dental insurance are assisted. Patients who need long-term payments to be able to go ahead with treatment are offered either a bank card, a healthcare financing program or an electronic fund transfer.

Work together, as a team, to determine your financial policy. Get comfortable with presenting the options. Know that your patients' comfort with the policy will be a direct reflection of your own comfort.

Promote bank cards to the fullest degree. Get involved with a healthcare financing program. Use the instruction in the upcoming chapters not only to learn how to present, but also how to build your practice with these programs. They are wonderful services for your patients, services that will lead to customer/patient satisfaction, increased new patient flow, and reduced cost of operation.

Becoming Involved with a Healthcare Financing Program: Getting Out of the Banking Business

"There's a way to do it better—find it!"
— THOMAS A. EDISON

U nderstanding the credit business as it applies to dentistry may be a tedious study. However, clarity in this vital part of your practice will help you to make the following decisions:

- To get out of the banking business and not look back.

- Reduce the amount of money you are spending on the statement and collection portion of your practice.

- Get involved with a healthcare financing program. (ASAP)

- Be more confident in presenting the program to your patients.

- Build your practice without increasing the overhead in the area of financial management.

COST OF CREDIT

In the following section, I will outline the cost of carrying accounts on your own books. The figures in the illustrations that accompany these pages are not important. The percentages are what makes the difference.

The accompanying illustration represents a $200,000 practice. You will need to multiply the figures to make them appropriate for your own practice.

The average dental practice receives approximately 50% of its revenue in the form of insurance checks If a dental practice has a gross annual income of $200,000 that would mean approximately $100,000 of that practice's revenue would be coming from insurance reimbursement.

About 30% of the income for most dental practices comes from cash or check. For a $200,000 practice that means that about $60,000 of income is generated by cash across the counter.

This leaves a remaining 20% that is the credit business, the credit portion of the practice or the billed charges portion of the business. Those are the people with whom you make financial agreements to make payments directly to the practice. These are the people to whom you begin sending statements and doing your own collections—your private pay accounts receivable. In our example of the $200,000 practice, this represents approximately $40,000 worth of yearly revenue.

The ADA tells us that the average practice in the U.S. collects approximately 96%. This means that the average dental practice is writing off about 4% or suffers a 4% loss. You may think that is not too bad—96% collection, or a 4% loss—not bad. (Fig. 2–1)

Well, let's look at that 4% loss and really look at it with open eyes. It becomes important to identify where the loss is coming from and what that loss really means to the profitability of your practice.

Go back to that average $200,000 practice that is experiencing a 4% write off. Four percent of 200,000 is $8000. This dentist wrote off $8000. Now answer these questions. Did the loss come from the $100,000 that was insurance? I doubt it. You may have a little bit of difficulty getting a quick turn around on insurance. But you do receive payment. Does the 4% loss come from the

Tips To Bank On

The ADA tells us that the average practice in the U.S. collects approximately 96%.

Value Analysis Example

- Annual Gross Revenue $200,000
  Insurance (50%) $100,000
  Cash (30%) $60,000
- Billed Charges (20%) $40,000
- Uncollected Revenue – % of Gross 4%
  % of Billed Charges 20%
- Statements Per Month 200
- Average American Dental Practice Collects 96%

© *Dr. T. Warren Center*

Figure 2–1

portion of the practice that is cash across the counter? Probably not. You may have a check bounce every once in a while, but that is not going to have a strong effect on your percentages.

So, if the loss did not come from insurance and it did not come from cash across the counter, there is only one place from which the loss could have come. That is the portion of the practice where you are carrying accounts for patients.

People may not intend to become past due with their accounts. A patient may say, "I will pay you $100 a month". Then that becomes difficult for them and they begin to pay $50 a month. Then something happens and that becomes $20 a month. Then they may miss a month or two and well, you can see that the account that you thought was going to be a three-month account, is now a six, nine, 12-month account, or you don't collect it at all.

Another interesting fact learned from the world of finance is that when an average family receives a check at the end of the month, that family pays bills in the following manner. First, a family pays the house payment, followed by utilities and food; then, a car payment (if there is one). A fourth payment is plastic. The dentist is number 35 out of 36.

Therefore. we know that if a family is having some difficulty making ends meet that it *might not be* that the dentist is a payment priority. I'm not saying that this is good, I'm just saying that this is the way it is. That is why the majority of loss experienced over a year is from the credit portion of your business.

Let's look closer at that loss. We agree that the entire $8000 is coming from the $40,000 that is being carried on the practice's books. The $8000 is 20% of the $40,000 credit business. In essence, this practice is having a 4% total loss of revenue but is having a 20% loss in its credit business. This is an incredibly important fact to realize. There is approximately a 20% loss coming from the credit portion of the average dental practice.

DIRECT COST OF BILLING AND COLLECTING

Let's take this one step further and analyze how much it is costing you, in terms of overhead, to run a credit business within your own practice. If you are sending an average of 200 statements a month, you're going to be investing approximately $1700 in materials alone—stamps, envelopes, statements, pegboard or computer materials, etc. If you send 200 statements a month and you are paying a person $6 an hour to handle this portion of your practice, and if this person is preparing one statement per minute, you are investing approximately $4600 per year in the labor costs of preparing and sending statements and in time invested in collection management—if collection is being done.

In addition, you are probably doing some collection calls. Based on a very conservative $15 a month for long distance calls, that is $190 per year in telephone expense. Adding these costs together, the statement and collection portion of your practice costs approximately $6,490—labor, materials, and management. The cost of billing and collecting is $6,490 minimum. That's 16.2% of the credit portion of your practice. (Fig. 2–2)

Direct Cost of Billing and Collecting

- Materials $1,700 yr.

- Labor $4,600 yr.

- Long Distance Calls $190 yr.

- Total $6,490 yrs.

16.2 of Billed Charges

© Dr. T. Warren Center

Figure 2–2

RECEIVABLE MANAGEMENT COSTS

There is another cost that goes along with managing accounts receivable. In addition to the $8000 in write-offs, there is one more loss. The world of banking tells us that for every month that an account sits on your own books doing nothing for you that it loses approximately 1% of its worth—or a 12% loss over the year. This is called "the loss of the dollar". If you have an average of $20,000 per month on your books in accounts receivable, you are going to be losing about 12% of the worth of that money over a year—1% per month. Twelve percent of an average of $20,000 in accounts receivable is a $2400 loss over a year.

If you could have had that money in hand, you could have either invested it or serviced debts. Then your money would have been working for you rather than decreasing in value.

Let's add all of that up. Remember, this practice had an $8000 loss from write-off of uncollectibles. Now we see that there is a $2400 "loss of the dollar". That equals $10,400. That's now 26% of the credit portion of your practice. (Fig. 2–3)

A $10,400 figure in receivables management plus the $6490 direct cost of billing and collecting equals $16,890. That is how much it costs a $200,000 practice to run a credit business over a

---

Receivables Management Cost

- Accounts Receivable $2,400 yr.
  12% of 20,000

- Uncollected Revenue $8,000 yr.
  20% of $40,000

- Total Receivable Management   _____
  Cost for Billed Charges $10,400 yr.

26% of Billed Charges

© Dr. T. Warren Center

Figure 2–3

year's period of time. What percentage is $16,890 of the $40,000 credit business? $16,890 is 42.2% of this practice's credit business. (Fig. 2–4)

Let that soak in just a minute—42.2% . The average general dental practice has an overhead of between 60 to 65%. If it costs 42.2% to manage the credit aspect of the practice and the overhead of the practice is 60–65%, guess what? You're breaking even or going in the hole, on the portion of your practice that is credit business. That makes no sense.

Get out of the banking business. Put the banking aspect or the credit aspect of your business into the hands of professionals, professional people who spend every day working with patients and their accounts. These specialists who are managing the healthcare financing programs have the professional ability to collect gently but firmly with the persistence that must be applied to obtain effective collection.

Again, referring to the American Dental Association, approximately 50% of the people in the United States are not even going to the dentist. There are four main reasons that people do not seek dental care or do not say "yes" to the treatment that the dentist is recommending:

1. Lack dental education. No perceived need.

2. Fear of the cost. "It costs too much"; "I can't afford it".

Total Cost of Billed Charges

- Direct Billing and Collecting $6,490 yr.

- Accounts Receivable Management $10,400 yr.

- Total $16,890 yr.

42.2 of Billed Revenue

© *Dr. T. Warren Center*

Figure 2–4

3. Fear of the dentistry itself. Apprehension.

4. Time—"it is not convenient". It is more and more difficult for people to leave work for dental appointments.

Offering a healthcare financing program will help both you and your patients deal with Fear of Cost. Patients will be able to accept treatment that otherwise might be rejected or delayed. You will be able to increase production significantly because of your ability to overcome the barrier of cost. Both parties win.

Also, if you are able to accomplish more dentistry per appointment and see the patient for fewer visits, that helps both parties to deal with the real issue of "time"

The available healthcare financing programs are different in protocol, but the vast majority of them are going to have a service charge. That service charge ranges from about 4% to 15%. Many practitioners think "Oh, no, that's terrible. That's too much. I'm not going to pay that much."

However, look at this is a new light. By carrying accounts on your own books it is costing you approximately 42.2%. You don't even have to put a pencil to it to realize that if a company will handle or manage the credit aspect of your practice for anywhere from 4 to 15% that you are saving an incredible

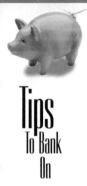

"A penny saved

is a

penny earned."

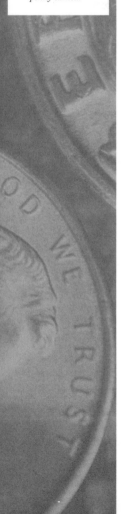

amount of money in overhead. Instead of 42.2%, it is going to cost you 4% to 15%.

This is essential in a dental practice where overhead is climbing on a regular basis. It doesn't make any sense to try to increase the productivity in the practice without watching the overhead as well. Then, and only then, can you begin to realize profitability. It's not how much you produce that makes the difference, it's how much you keep.

How Do These Programs Work?

When you have diagnosed some necessary or desired treatment and are discussing the financial responsibility, payment options will be discussed. If a person indicates that he/she needs to make small payments and spread those payments out over a period of time, you would introduce your financing program.

Example: "Ms. Jones, I understand that you feel concerned about the investment you will be making. Many of our patients have felt the same concern until they found out that we do offer long-term financing in our practice. We have a financial partner, ABC Financing Company. You complete an application right here in our practice—you don't have to go anywhere. Once you have completed the application, we can send or fax it to the company to see about establishing a line of credit for you. Once that line of credit is established, we can begin your treatment. You will then be able to make small monthly payments and spread the payments over a long period of time. You will only be required to make a minimum payment each month. Dr. Jameson has paid all necessary fees for you to become involved and there is no annual fee. Therefore, you only pay for the service when you use it."

Once the patient is extended a line of credit, you will finance their dentistry as the treatment proceeds. A charge slip is filled out as service is rendered. Those slips are then sent to the company for processing, or are sent by electronic means directly to the company. Then, you will receive payment for the services that you have provided, minus the service fee. The patient begins making payments to the financing program. They no longer owe the dentist. If the patient defaults on the account for any reason at all, the dentist is no way, shape, or form, responsible for the account ever again. The programs are non-recourse and place the dentist at no risk whatsoever.

Remember, the scenario of the $200,000 practice? Historically, dental practices have been writing off approximately 20% of the credit portion of their revenues. But if you allow a professional financing company to handle that portion of your practice—the credit portion—you will not experience that kind of loss.

Example: Take a $1000 charge, and let's say the service fee is 5%. You would receive a check for $950. That would be the end of that. You would not send statements. You would not handle collection issues. You would receive your money. The service fee is, in essence, the salary you are paying the company to work for you. They are your financial partner and teammate. These are excellent programs and deserve your careful study and attention.

Offering this type of financing will expand your ability to serve people. Your increase in production would probably be anywhere from 10 to 30%. Why? Because there is a portion of the population that needs this type of financing in order to make a major investment, like a $500 dental treatment. You will be saving money in cost of operation in the credit aspect of your practice, plus you will be making it possible for a portion of your patient family to go ahead with treatment that would not otherwise be able to do so.

So many dentists say that they have more dentistry sitting in their charts than they have ever provided. Offering this type of program will get some of that dentistry out of the charts and into the mouths of your patients.

The American Dental Association says that for every 10 years that a dentist provides dental care, that he/she has approximately $1,000,000 worth of dentistry that has been diagnosed but remains undone. Approximately $100,000 per year.

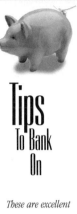

Tips
To Bank
On

These are excellent programs and deserve your careful study and attention.

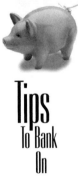

Tips
To Bank
On

So many dentists say that they have more dentistry sitting in their charts than they have ever provided.

In our own dental practice, we place approximately $100,000 of dental care *per year* on our financing program. My dentist husband, John, believes that this would be $100,000 worth of dental treatment that he would not otherwise be able to provide. We feel that there are many people who are receiving excellent care who would not have been able to do so if we were not making this option available to them. He is not one of those statistics that says that he has $1,000,000 worth of dentistry sitting in his charts. In the first 10 years that we participated with a healthcare financing program, we placed $1,000,000 on that program.

BENEFITS

- Increase productivity to make optimum, quality dentistry affordable for the vast majority of your patients.

- Invest less money in running a credit business.

- Maximize time for your staff.

- Instead of spending lots of time preparing and sending statements and handling collections, team members can turn their attention to practice building and patient care.

That's how you build a practice. You focus on giving patients all that they expect—and a little bit more each and every time.

SUMMARY

Many dentists have understood the benefit of becoming involved with these programs. However, they think that the programs don't work. They can't get people to accept the program, they don't see practice growth as a result of using the program, and they become frustrated.

Your success with one of these programs will be in direct proportion to the confidence of the team members in the program, how they present the program, and how actively you market the program. I'm not sure that the programs don't work for those practices—I think those practices don't work with the programs.

In the next chapter, we will study six ways to maximize a healthcare financing program. These six ways will make a 10-30% positive difference in your practice. These six programs have proven to be effective and powerful in practices throughout the country and the world for those who have followed our instructions. You can do the same thing.

Maximizing a Healthcare Financing Program: Building Your Practice by Defusing the Fear of Cost

*"There is only one boss.
The customer. And he can fire everyone
in the company from the chairman on down,
simply by spending his money somewhere else."*

— SAM WALTON,
FOUNDER, WAL-MART STORES, INC.

So, you've become involved with a healthcare financing program, but you're not quite sure what to do with it. You expected to see some practice growth and some financial reward from the program, but that isn't happening yet. You're wondering what you can do to achieve both of these goals: practice growth and financial reward.

In this chapter, I will explain six ways to develop your practice using a healthcare financing program. In addition, I will suggest some verbal skills for explaining the program and for defusing some of the objections your patients will express about the program.

If you will follow the program as outlined, you can increase revenues in your practice anywhere from 10% to 30%. Where is your production right now? Would a 10% increase make a difference for you? Give the following ideas a try. They work!!

INTRODUCE THE PROGRAM TO YOUR ENTIRE PATIENT FAMILY

In a special mailing, or in your regularly published patient education newsletter, tell your existing patient family about the program. Present the program in an exciting, informative manner—one that stresses the benefits to the patient. (Fig. 3-1)

There's the key. Point out how the program will benefit the patient and/or the patient's family. Do not stress how much it will benefit you.

In this special mailing include a brochure about the program; some offices include an application. Make it easy for the patient to become involved.

Some patients in your practice will not need the program. If they don't need financial assistance, they won't apply. However, some people may not be coming to you on a regular basis or may be putting off needed or desired treatment because of the *fear of cost*. Others may have completed one phase of treatment but do not want to schedule the next phase of treatment because they *owe you money*. If this is the case, establishing a line of credit may break the cost barrier. If they owe the financing program instead of you, they may be more willing and able to go ahead with treatment.

Get the program into the hands of *your* consumers—the patients.

Remember the number one reason that people do not come to the dentist is that there is no perceived need and the number two reason is that of the fear of cost. Introducing a patient to the Healthcare Financing Program via a newsletter works to relieve both of those barriers. This newsletter serves to educate people

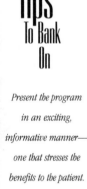

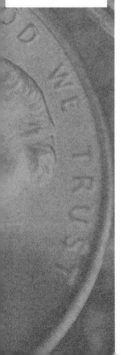

Tips
To Bank On

Present the program

in an exciting,

informative manner—

one that stresses the

benefits to the patient.

Dear Friends,

It is with great pleasure that I introduce to you a new method of financing for healthcare that we are offering in our office. The company behind this method of financing is called (Name). I would like to explain briefly what this is, how it works, and what benefits it has for you.

(Name) is a company that offers convenient financing for dental care. A person or family applies for the program in our office. It is very easy to apply and the acceptance rate is very high. The patient can then finance any dental treatment. You may spread your payments over a long period of time and keep the monthly payments quite small. If you choose to pay the balance off early, there is no penalty. It is a *revolving payment plan*—every time you make a payment, your next one is smaller. This is a positive and revolutionary addition to the healthcare field and is sweeping the country.

In your office we have found that our patients who are using the program are reaping many benefits, such as the following:

(1) Convenient and regular monthly payments—easily budgeted.

(2) Long term pay out.

(3) No large payments due at one time.

(4) Balance of your insurance can be financed and then easily budgeted.

(5) Necessary treatment does not have to be put off due to financial problems.

(6) Continuous Care appointments for the family can become more regular—thus insuring proper dental care for all members of the family.

(7) Emergency treatment does not have to be ignored or "financially fearful".

We offer quality service to our patients both dentally and

Figure 3–1 Special mailing—new finance program.

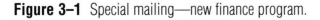

personally—because we care so much for all of you. Now we feel that we can come full circle in serving you by offering a financial plan that also meets your needs.

Enclosed you will find a brochure that explains the program and an application form. If you are interested, fill out the application in full and mail it or bring it to our office. If you are already a member of (Name), please pass this application and brochure on to a friend or relative.

If you have any questions at all, or if we can help you in any way, please don't hesitate to call the office. We are here to help you—always.

Yours for better dental health,

John H. Jameson, D.D.S.

Figure 3–1 *(Continued)*

about the value of dentistry as well as the new options available in dentistry today.

Practices spend a great deal of time nurturing a new patient flow. Spending time nurturing the existing patient family makes a great deal of sense. Most practices can double from within if time and effort is spent on reactivation and retention. I'm not saying that you don't want to nurture a new patient flow. Obviously, you do. But I encourage you to maximize your market share by dealing with the patient families that you already have existing in your files.

NEWSLETTERS

Newsletters? Are they effective? Many marketing specialists and I believe that they are. Many practices say that they can't afford to do a newsletter. Or that they don't have time to do a newsletter. Again, remember that the lack of dental education is the number one reason that people don't receive dentistry. They either don't come in or they don't say "yes" to the dentistry that you recommend. And, thus, your main commission as dental professionals is to be educators. One of the very best ways to educate your patient family—next to your in-office one-on-one education—is through the patient newsletter.

Let me quickly suggest to you a way of doing a newsletter. We produce a quarterly newsletter, and have produced newsletters for over 10 years. This newsletter serves many purposes:

1. We want to be in the homes of our patient families in a positive way on a regular basis. When they think of the dentist we want them to think of the dentist in a positive way. When they think of the dentist, we hope that they think of our practice.

2. We want to inform our patients of various aspects of dentistry in an effort to soothe anxieties and any questions about certain procedures. We want them to know what is happening in dentistry. Sometimes we assume that all patients in the world know about the exciting things that are happening in dentistry. They don't. It is our commission to educate them about the new advances in dentistry.

3. We want to let our patient family know what we are doing in our practice to keep abreast of the latest and best in health care for their benefit.

4. We want to express our appreciation for their confidence in us.

5. We invite them to refer their family and friends to us.

Your newsletter needs to be economical and efficient both in time and in money. So the following is a way that you might do this and serve both the essential requirements. By a designated day in the month, say the 15th, the dentist and the team members have written or gathered data for the newsletter. By the 15th of the month all the necessary information should be in the hands of a specific person who is going to type or cut and paste the information for the newsletter. We might see an article or just a brief bit of information that is appropriate for our patient family. We cut out that information and utilize it in the newsletter. Many times if we want to reprint an article from the American Cancer Association or American Heart Association, we will contact them for their permission. They are thrilled. They say "Our purpose is to educate people and if you can do that— please do. All we ask is that you send us a copy of your newsletter." So we do.

We use a legal size piece of paper front and back. We take this typed copy with cut and pasted information to a printer. The printer keeps our logo on file. They not only print the newsletter for us, but they return it to us tri-folded. On one side of this tri-folded piece of legal size paper, they print our return address, our bulk permit number, and address correction requested. The bulk rate mailing permit costs about $80 a year. For that you can mail for approximately half the normal mailing rates. You must mail in volume of 200 or more. So you can see that the bulk mailing number pays for itself very quickly. Now I will tell you that if you mail with a bulk mail permit, you must put your newsletters in zip code order, and that is not easy. At a staff meeting the team all gathers together over lunch and labels and zip codes the newsletters. "Many hands make light work." We found in one or two hours we can get this task accomplished. You can have a good time doing it together. Or, hire a high school student to come one time per quarter for this project. (Fig. 3–2)

We are computerized so we just have our computer spit out the labels and that's no big deal. For those of you who are not computerized, let me tell you a cost- and time-effective way to do a set of labels for you families. Go to your office supply and buy a box of labels. There are 33 labels to the page, or three rows of 11 labels. I suggest you go to a high school and hire a business student to come for a couple of hours after school for a week. Pay them minimum wage and have them type a label for each one of your patient families. Then slip that master into a plastic cover and threaten the life of anybody who ever touches it again. Because this is your master and you don't want

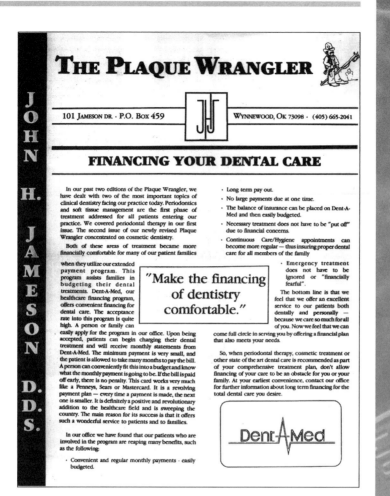

THE PLAQUE WRANGLER

101 JAMESON DR. · P.O. BOX 459   WYNNEWOOD, OK 73098 · (405) 665-2041

FINANCING YOUR DENTAL CARE

In our past two editions of the Plaque Wrangler, we have dealt with two of the most important topics of clinical dentistry facing our practice today. Periodontics and soft tissue management are the first phase of treatment addressed for all patients entering our practice. We covered periodontal therapy in our first issue. The second issue of our newly revised Plaque Wrangler concentrated on cosmetic dentistry.

Both of these areas of treatment became more financially comfortable for many of our patient families when they utilize our extended payment program. This program assists families in budgeting their dental treatments. Dent-A-Med, our healthcare financing program, offers convenient financing for dental care. The acceptance rate into this program is quite high. A person or family can easily apply for the program in our office. Upon being accepted, patients can begin charging their dental treatment and will receive monthly statements from Dent-A-Med. The minimum payment is very small, and the patient is allowed to take many months to pay the bill. A person can conveniently fit this into a budget and know what the monthly payment is going to be. If the bill is paid off early, there is no penalty. This card works very much like a Penneys, Sears or Mastercard. It is a revolving payment plan — every time a payment is made, the next one is smaller. It is definitely a positive and revolutionary addition to the healthcare field and is sweeping the country. The main reason for its success is that it offers such a wonderful service to patients and to families.

In our office we have found that our patients who are involved in the program are reaping many benefits, such as the following:

· Convenient and regular monthly payments - easily budgeted.

· Long term pay out.
· No large payments due at one time.
· The balance of insurance can be placed on Dent-A-Med and then easily budgeted.
· Necessary treatment does not have to be "put off" due to financial concerns.
· Continuous Care/Hygiene appointments can become more regular — thus insuring proper dental care for all members of the family
· Emergency treatment does not have to be ignored or "financially fearful".

> "Make the financing of dentistry comfortable."

The bottom line is that we feel that we offer an excellent service to our patients both dentally and personally — because we care so much for all of you. Now we feel that we can come full circle in serving you by offering a financial plan that also meets your needs.

So, when periodontal therapy, cosmetic treatment or other state of the art dental care is recommended as part of your comprehensive treatment plan, don't allow financing of your care to be an obstacle for you or your family. At your earliest convenience, contact our office for further information about long term financing for the total dental care you desire.

Dent-A-Med

Figure 3–2 Patient Education Newsletter

to have to do it again. When it comes time to print your labels, take that master, put it in your copy machine run a blank set of labels through the copy machine and you have a copy of labels for your patient families. Of course, every month you will be adding the new patients as they are added to your practice. This is a very easy and cost-effective way for you to get a very vital list of patient families that you can utilize in your marketing.

This is the way we do our newsletter. We produced one entire issue on the Healthcare Financing Program when we made our initial introduction of the program. Now every so often we reintroduce the fact that we do have financing available, just to keep that fresh in patients' minds.

In January of every year we remind our patients that a new year has begun and that this new year indicates a new maximum for their insurance. Therefore if they have incomplete treatment, or if they would like to come in for continuous care, or if there are people in their family who have not been able to come in to receive treatment, that this new year offers the opportunity to utilize their new insurance benefits. We encourage them to utilize this wonderful supplement to their healthcare. If they have dental insurance, they can finance the balance after the insurance pays or if they don't have dental insurance, this is a comfortable and convenient way to take care of the financing of their dentistry. We do this in January.

Also in October of every year we send a letter to our patients reminding them that if they have not utilized or taken advantage of their yearly maximum of their insurance, now is a good time to do that. (Fig. 3–3) If they have existing dentistry that needs to be completed, we encourage them to maximize their insurance benefits. Rather than to wait until the end of the year, a very hectic time, to call now to schedule an appointment for that dentistry. Again to maximize their insurance, we also tell them that if they have any concerns about the balance after insurance pays, we do have comfortable and convenient financing available for them.

So that is how we introduce our Healthcare Financing Program to our entire patient family. Bear in mind that when a new patient comes to the practice, one on one, we introduce the program enthusiastically to them. The very best way to market this service is for everyone in the office, everyone on the team, to understand the program, enlighten patients about it, be excited about it and to *offer it*.

I can tell you confidently that your new patient flow will increase as patients become involved with a financing program. People will go home and say, "Hey, my dentist has this new program available. You can finance your dentistry and pay it out. The payments are real small." Personal referrals will always be your best source for new patients, However, we have found that many patients are coming to us because they now know that we offer comfortable convenient long term financing. In our Yellow Page ad we also make note that we do offer convenient financing. About six to eight percent of new patients will come from a Yellow Page ad. If you utilize the Yellow Page ads, it is a good idea to let people know that you have comfortable financing available. (Fig. 3–4)

In addition, to the initial introduction of the program through a special mailing or a patient education newsletter, consider introducing the financial program, as well as your entire

---

ATTENTION!
INSURANCE COVERAGE
ENDING FOR YEAR

NOW is the time to plan for the completion of your dental treatment before the end of the year. All insurance plans have a yearly maximum. If you do not use this maximum amount—the remainder is lost.

IF you have already met your deductible, and you have treatment to be completed, or to be started—take advantage of your benefits this year. If necessary, we can use the maximum allowed this year, and complete the treatment next year with next year's allowance.

Good planning will allow you to take advantage of the full benefit of your policy. Please do not wait until the last few days of the year, when our contested schedule will make it difficult to appoint a convenient time for you.

OUR goal is to provide you with quality dental services. If we can help you maximize your dental insurance coverage in the process, we will be very pleased.

Please give us a call as soon as possible.

Sincerely,

Dr. John H. Jameson and Team

Insurance/End of Year

Figure 3–3

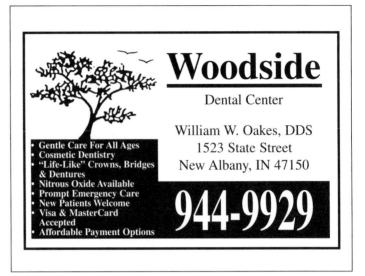

Figure 3–4 Telephone ad of my client and friend, Dr. Woody Oakes.

financial policy, to your patients through a practice brochure. (Fig. 3–5)

A practice brochure needs to be a marketing piece—a marketing piece that lets people know who you are, where you are, what you do, and what makes you *special*. In other words, it needs to *not* be a naggy, boring, ugly piece of literature (I use the term loosely) that gets thrown in the trash. Rather, it needs to be attractive, informational, and inviting.

One of the most inviting things that you can do is let new, or potentially new, patients know that they need not fear the cost of their dental treatment and that you have comfortable options available for payment.

Hey, folks, the financial options that I recommended earlier are a *service*. You are going out of your way to make the dental treatment affordable—dental treatment that you believe is vital to health and well being. Let people know that you do have this service available. Defuse the fear of cost in advance of a patient's entrance into your practice.

Also, on your patient information sheet, introduce your financial options. We send this information sheet/health history

WELCOME...

TO OUR DENTAL OFFICE

WELCOME AND SPECIAL! It is our goal to help you feel this way every time you call or come to our office. Your health, comfort, and individual needs are foremost in our minds.

THE PURPOSE of this brochure is to familiarize you with our office and to make you feel more at home. We hope that many questions you may have will be answered. However, please feel free to contact any member of our team — we're here for you.

WE ARE COMMITTED to excellence and to service in all areas of dental care. We are here to help you achieve and maintain good oral health for your lifetime.

PROFESSIONALISM
IS IMPORTANT...

- We stay current with the latest and best dental techniques and services by continuing our education on a regular basis.
- We practice excellent sterilization and infection control methods for your safety and protection.
- We provide the skills of periodontal therapists/dental hygienists to restore and maintain healthy gum tissue.
- Our staff of professionals is exceptionally qualified to provide expertise in each department within the office.

WE TREAT
OUR PATIENTS
WITH SPECIAL CARE...

THE PHILOSOPHY of our office is to provide optimum dentistry for our patients, in a caring and loving way.

PHYSICALLY...
EMOTIONALLY...
FINANCIALLY...

PHYSICALLY...
To make your dental care physically comfortable we offer audio analgesia (stereo headsets) and nitrous oxide analgesia. You can lay back, relax, and listen to your choice of music. Your dental appointment will fly by and you will be ready to go on with your day. We offer caring dentistry for adults and children.

EMOTIONALLY...
We know that your smile affects all areas of your life. Your smile affects your self confidence and greatly affects your appearance. Therefore, we do our best to listen to your particular needs and strive to meet those needs. We can help you achieve the smile you've always wanted. Ask about our COSMETIC DENTISTRY.

FINANCIALLY...
To make your dental care financially comfortable our office offers a variety of payment options.
1) Cash, personal checks
2) 5% cash courtesy for advance payment of entire treatment plan
3) VISA/Mastercard
4) Insurance on assignment
5) Long-term or regular monthly payments are available through our extended payment plan — Dent-A-Med.

DENTAL SERVICES
AVAILABLE...

Dr. Jameson has extensive training in all areas of general dentistry.

RESTORATIVE
AND
COSMETIC DENTISTRY

- Bonding
- Porcelain Veneers
- Cosmetic Recontouring
- Crowns and Bridges
- Full and Partial Dentures

OTHER SERVICES

- Endodontics (root canals)
- Non-surgical Periodontal (gum disease) Therapy

SELECTED AREAS

- Oral Surgery
- Periodontal Surgery
- TMJ Treatment
- Dental Implants

PREVENTIVE DENTISTRY

- Dental Cleaning
- Oral Health Examinations
- Radiographs
- Sealants
- Fluoride Treatments

Before we recommend any type of treatment, we want to LISTEN to and UNDERSTAND your desires, your likes and dislikes, and your concerns about your dental care. Only then are we able to provide you with the excellent care you deserve.

Figure 3–5 Practice Brochure

to patients prior to their arrival in our office. This *welcome packet* includes the practice brochure, the information sheet/health history, a card confirming the appointment, a patient education newsletter, and information about our financing program. We send this to a patient as soon as he/she calls to schedule a new patient evaluation. We ask patients to complete their information sheet/health history and mail it back to us prior to their arrival so that we can be well prepared for their visit. All of the information will already be in the computer, so Dr. Jameson will be able to review their health history in advance of their appointment. We will be able to seat them much more quickly since all of the necessary paperwork will have been completed. (Fig. 3–6)

They see our financial policy on the brochure and on the information sheet. It is presented in a very positive way. There is no question or confusion. Everything is spelled out before the fact. No confusion. No "after the fact" information. Up front is the best way to deal with any arrangement. Dr. Burt Press has told us for a long time to "inform before you perform." That applies to the treatment to be rendered and to the financial

JOHN H. JAMESON, DDS
101 JAMESON DRIVE • P.O. BOX 459
WYNNEWOOD, OKLAHOMA 73098
(405) 665-2041

**PLEASE COMPLETE AND
RETURN TO FRONT DESK**

NAME:	Last	First			Middle	

| ADDRESS: | Street or P.O. Box# | City | State | Zip Code | PHONE NUMBER
HOME:
WORK: |
|---|---|---|---|---|---|

| AGE: Yrs. | BIRTH DATE | Mo. | Day | Year | BIRTHPLACE | ( ) Married
( ) Unmarried
( ) Separated | SOCIAL SECURITY NO. (if child, parent's)
DRIVER'S LICENSE NO. |
|---|---|---|---|---|---|---|---|

OCCUPATION	EMPLOYER		HOW LONG EMPLOYED	ADDRESS & PHONE NO.

| PERSON RESPONSIBLE FOR BILL
(if married, spouse's name) | | AGE | ADDRESS | RELATIONSHIP | SOCIAL SECURITY NO.
DRIVER'S LICENSE NO. |
|---|---|---|---|---|---|

OCCUPATION	EMPLOYER	HOW LONG EMPLOYED	ADDRESS & PHONE NO.

INSURANCE INFORMATION

INSURED PERSON'S FULL NAME

SOCIAL SECURITY NUMBER	RELATIONSHIP TO PATIENT	WORK PHONE

INSURANCE COMPANY NAME	GROUP OR UNION NAME	GROUP OR LOCAL NUMBER

EMPLOYER'S NAME	FULL ADDRESS OF EMPLOYER

GETTING TO KNOW YOU

1. Why did you select our office?_____

2. Whom may we thank for referring you?_____

3. Is another member of your family or relative a patient in our practice?

4. Person to contact for emergency:_____
Phone:_____

5. When was your last dental visit?_____
When was the last time you had complete dental X-rays taken?

6. Have you ever had any teeth removed?_____
How long have these teeth been missing?_____
Have these teeth been replaced?

How? ☐ Bridge ☐ Partial ☐ Denture ☐ Implants

PAYMENT ALTERNATIVES

Please check appropriate box:

☐ 1. Cash and personal checks are accepted as your treatments are provided.

☐ 2. As a special service to you, we will give you a five percent (5X) cash courtesy if you pay for your entire treatment plan in full, in advance.

☐ 3. If you have dental insurance, we want you to receive the full benefit of it. Our office staff can assist you in completing your insurance forms and verifying the coverage that your particular program provides. We accept assignment of your insurance payment; another service to you.

This means that you are responsible for your deductible and the portion the insurance does not cover when you see the doctor. Remember, however, that you are responsible for the account if the insurance company, for any reason, does not honor their commitment to you and to us.

☐ 4. Mastercard, Visa and Discover.

☐ 5. For those of you needing an extended payment program, our office offers Dent-A-Med, which, when you are accepted, will allow extended small monthly payments for the treatment received. This is a health care financing program.

FOR ALL PATIENTS

I hereby authorize the doctor to perform any and all forms of treatment, medication, and therapy, that may be indicated in connection with the dental care of the patient above and further authorize and consent that the doctor chooses and employs such assistance as he deems fit. I also understand that previous to treatment, full explanation of the procedure(s) involved will be given by the doctor and/or his staff. I agree to pay for all services rendered by this office.

SIGNATURE OF RESPONSIBLE PARTY	RELATIONSHIP	DATE	©1985 JAMESON MANAGEMENT GROUP

Figure 3-6

responsibility. We inform patients of the financial options right from the start. People are glad to know that there are options available for most any financial situation.

Remember that repetition is the key to learning and the key to getting good results from your marketing efforts. Do not introduce your financial policy or your healthcare financing program once and expect it to be readily accepted. It won't be. You must repetitively reintroduce the programs to your patients, via newsletters, mailings, telephone ad, newspaper articles, and verbal introduction during the financial presentation.

ACCOUNTS RECEIVABLE TRANSFER

As was illustrated in the previous chapter, every day that an account sits on your books doing nothing, you lose money because of (1) the cost of operation for running a banking business within your practice; (2) the chances of never collecting the account; and (3) the "loss of the dollar" as it sits on your books depreciating in value make the carrying of accounts a difficult business process.

Therefore, consider making an active effort to transfer as many of your existing accounts as possible to your healthcare financing program.

SUGGESTED STEPS FOR THIS TRANSFER:

1. Analyze your accounts receivable. Determine the following:

    a. How much is insurance? How much is private pay?

    b. Of the private pay accounts, how many are 30, 60, 90, 120 *(or more)* days past due?

    c. Those accounts that are extremely past due and have had no activity whatsoever, may need to be turned over for legal action. (Make sure that the dentist approves all accounts to be *turned over* or *written off*).

2. For all of the remaining accounts, create a letter introducing the idea of transferring accounts to the Healthcare Financing Program. (Fig. 3–7) Expound on the benefits of the program, such as:

    a. Longer time in which to pay the account.

    b. Smaller monthly payments.

    c. No large payments due at one time.

Name
Street
City, State, Zip

Dear (Name):

Our office has found that we must constantly keep abreast of the latest dental advances in order to offer our patients the best clinical care possible. We also search for new methods of payment which will allow our patients to receive the necessary care when needed or desired. We have recently accessed a new financial partner who works with us to make the financing of our patients' dental care comfortable.

Enclosed is an informational brochure and an application for (Name of the company). This company works with us to offer an extended payment plan to our patients—a plan that lets you receive the necessary treatment, finance that treatment, and spread the payments out over your desired length of time—keeping your monthly payments small and convenient.

One month from the postmark of this letter, we will be forced to initiate a service fee of 1.75% per month for any past due accounts. If you have an outstanding balance with our practice, you can transfer your existing balance to (name of company) and the service fee is lower. The service for (name of company) is 1.625% per month which is lower than ours. In addition, if you transfer your balance, your monthly payments will be smaller and you can take longer to pay.

This is a great program that gives you tremendous benefits. You simply complete the enclosed application and send it or bring it to the office. We will send it to the company for processing and then, once you have received a line of credit, we will transfer your existing balance. Easy. Simple. Beneficial.

In the future, should you or a member of your family need dental care, you will not have to worry about *putting* off that care. You will have a line of credit established for yourself and your family and it

Figure 3–7 Initial Accounts Receivable Transfer Letter

will be there when you need it. You do not pay anything for this service. Dr. Jameson has paid all necessary fees for you to become involved. In addition, there is no yearly fee. So, you only pay for it when you use it.

If you have any questions, please feel free to call our office. We feel that this breakthrough is what our patients have been looking for in dental financing.

Sincerely,

John H. Jameson, D.D.S. & Team

Special Offer: If you pay off your balance within 30 days of the postmark of this letter, we will give you 10% off your existing balance.

Figure 3–7 *(Continued)*

  d. No initial or yearly fee to become involved with the program.

  e. Available credit for emergencies or for necessary and desired treatment.

  f. If you are charging a service fee and it is more than the financing program, in the letter let the patients know that the service fee for the financing program is lower. (If it is!)

 3. Send an application and a brochure with this letter. Send this letter in a separate mailing, rather than with statements. Place the letter on your letterhead stationery and place it in one of your letterhead envelopes. This needs to be a special mailing in order to get a special response from your patients.

You may wish to offer a 10% courtesy if the guarantor comes in and pays his/her balance in full within 30 days of the postmark of the letter. This, in itself, may bring in a great number of payments. (The cost of carrying the account on your own books will be greater than the courtesy given.)

4. At the next statement run—another month has passed—send a follow-up letter with another brochure and another application. (Remember that repetition is the key to learning). Let your patients know that you are serious about this service. (Fig. 3–8)

   In this letter let your patients know that you have changed accounting methods and are offering this financial service to those who wish to extend their payments over a long period of time. Remember to stress the benefits of the program and the benefits to the individuals.

5. Following the next statement run (you are now approximately 90 days into your accounts receivable transfer) begin a telephone campaign to all of those patients who have not responded to either one of your mailings. (Fig. 3–9)

   Track your telephone calls. Make notes of who you have called, those who were sent an application, the date you sent the application, the date it was received back in the office, and any comments relative to the conversation. (Fig. 3–10)

6. By the next statement run you should have had a strong response to your efforts—especially if you have followed the regime carefully and with commitment. If you are not going to follow the campaign through to the end—with consistency—don't expect a great response.

Many offices with whom I have worked have converted half of their accounts receivable to cash in a four-to six-month period of time. *Results are in direct correlation to effort put forth.*

Tips To Bank On

Results are in direct correlation to effort put forth.

Name
Street
City-State-Zip

Dear (Name):

Last month we introduced a new concept in healthcare financing. The program is called (Name of Company). You have received information regarding this innovative program. We have had an overwhelming response to this convenient method of financing dentistry from our patient friends.

In order to maintain comfortable fees for our patients, our accountant has insisted that we remove ourselves from the banking business. We have found that it is not time- or cost-efficient to run a banking business within our practice. And so, we have become involved with a healthcare financing program that will allow our patients to have smaller payments that can extend over a longer period of time.

The financial arrangements that we had previously made with you seem to have been difficult. Since the time of our arrangement, there have been occasions when the agreed payments were not made. Since this agreement has become difficult for you to maintain, we would like to encourage you to transfer your existing balance to (Name of Company). This could allow you to lower your monthly payments and would give you a longer time in which to pay.

We have enclosed a brochure about the program and an application. We would encourage you to study this information and to call our office with any questions. Complete the application and bring or mail it to our office. We will send the application to the company for processing. Once you are extended a line of credit, we will transfer your balance to (Name of Company).

We look forward to working with you to comfortably convert this account to a method of payment that would be more acceptable to you.

Sincerely,

Financial Coordinator

Figure 3–8 Letter #2 Accounts Receivable Transfer.

Telephone Campaign Script
Accounts Receivable Transfer

Business Manager: "Good Morning, Mrs. Jones. This is Cathy from Dr. Jameson's office. Mrs. Jones, last month we mailed some information about a new healthcare financing program that we have available in our office. Did you receive that information?

You did? Good. Mrs. Jones, my records indicate you have a balance with our practice of $_____. Mrs. Jones, we have found that many of our patients are more comfortable with smaller monthly payments that will fit more easily into their monthly budgets. These monthly payments can be spread out over a longer period of time.

Mrs. Jones, if you were to apply and be extended a line of credit with (Name of Company) we could immediately convert your account and your first monthly payment would be approximately $_____. Does this sound like a program that would be of interest to you?

Good. Can you come by the office today to fill out an application? Great! (Offer to send the application to her home if she cannot come in). We can send it in today, and once you receive a line of credit we will make the necessary conversion of your account.

Mrs. Jones, we want you to know how much we appreciate your cooperation. We believe that this is one of the best financial services we have been able to offer our patients."

Figure 3–9 Script for telephone calls for Accounts Receivable Transfer.

Note: If a patient is abiding by a previously agreed upon financial arrangement go ahead and offer the program to him/her, but willingly allow him/her to maintain this agreement if it is comfortable.

A good rule of thumb is to have no more than one times your average monthly production in accounts receivable, and

ACCOUNTS RECEIVABLES TRANSFER

DATE CONTACTED	PATIENT	PHONE	BAL.	LAST PAYMENT	HCFP	DATE APPLICATION SENT	RECEIVED	COMMENTS
1/17	Stephanie Jones	374-5289	$1000	10/93	$50/mo.	1/17	1/22	Glad to transfer balance
1/17	Mike Allen	374-7386	$562	11/93	$37/mo.	1/17		
1/17	Carrol Samuels	278-7439	$754	9/93	$45/mo.	1/17	1/30	Transferred balance

Figure 3–10 Tracking devices for Accounts Receivable Transfer.

that should be, mostly insurance turnaround. If you are electronically processing your claims the turnaround of claims will be significantly less than 30 days. The goal of a one month average of production on your accounts receivable may be less than you have heard in the past. The understanding of the cost of money and the understanding that the longer an account sits on your books the more difficult it is to collect has reduced that goal.

If you do have accounts receivable at the present time and if you feel that the outstanding amount is too great, perform an accounts receivable transfer. The money you have been carrying on your own books is going to be converted to cash and that doesn't hurt when bills have to be paid. The money sitting on your books is doing nothing but losing money for you every day. Conversion of these accounts is excellent business. The team is going to love the accounts receivable transfer, because they are going to get out of the statement and collection business. This gives them more time to take care of other necessary duties within the practice.

Most people are not crazy about sending 200–300 statements a month, analyzing those accounts and then doing the necessary collection calls, sending collection letters, etceteras. Most dental auxiliary would rather be doing marketing, public relations, handling insurance, or engineering the appointment book. Patients are thrilled with the accounts receivable transfer because most patients would rather owe a financing institution than to owe the dentist. In addition, their payments will probably be less per month.

We have *no* private pay accounts receivable in our own practice. We make arrangements with the patient to either take care of the payment in full before treatment begins and we give that patient a 5% accounting reduction if they choose to do this. We accept payment by the appointment with cash, check, or bank card. We also take insurance on assignment—carefully doing our best to maximize the insurance benefits for our patients, And for any long term or extended payments we offer our Healthcare Financing Program. From the time we initiated this policy, it was like putting a dam in the river called accounts receivable. From that point forward we no longer offered financing on our own books. Then we had to go through the process of cleaning up the mess of existing accounts receivable. We did this very successfully. The practices with whom we consult have found that they get the same results. Our consulting practices get out of the banking business.

Does this hurt productivity? No! All practices increase production significantly and certainly become more profitable. In addition, stress is relieved because the money from production is in the bank and is not sitting out there doing nothing. More time is available for the important activities that build the practice—time is not spent on statements and collection.

Many dentists have said to me, "I am concerned that some patients will be upset with me. I have been carrying accounts for so long that they might get upset and leave."

My experience has been this: Once you have set a financial policy and your patients understand it's to serve them better—to offer top quality dentistry at comfortable fees—they will be fine. Let them know that you had to get out of the banking business because it was not financially feasible for you to run a banking business within your practice. Maintain your commitment to quality. They will respect this. Presented in this manner I find that very few people become disgruntled. (Please re-examine Fig. 1–3.) They understand what you need to do and why. If you have focused your practice on offering quality service, they really won't want to go anywhere else or have any other dentist actively involved in their care. They will abide by your policy. They will understand and respect your request.

So that is accounts receivable transfer. I recommend that you follow this program. Take the concept and individualize it to fit you. No two practices are alike but these concepts will fit any practice—you just have to fine tune them to make them your own.

CHART AUDITING

Most dentists will agree that there is more dentistry sitting in their charts waiting to be done than they have ever done in their practicing days. We now know that one of the main reasons that people do not proceed with dental care is the "fear of cost". Therefore, going through all of the charts to reactivate people into the practice or to reinforce the need for the dental treatment can be a super practice builder—especially when this effort is combined with the introduction of your healthcare financing program.

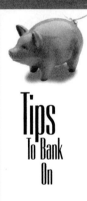

Tips To Bank On

. . . one of the main reasons that people do not proceed with dental care is the "fear of cost".

Suggested Procedure.

1. Decide how many charts are going to be audited per week (i.e., Two per day for a total of 8 or 10 per week). (Fig. 3–11) Gather the following information on each patient:

   - Last date seen

   - Last date of a cleaning and evaluation

Goals And Objectives

Goal:

Objective	Responsible Person	Time Frame	Evaluation
1. Start with A's. Audit 20 charts a week.	Jan	20 Charts per week	Week #1 -- 25 Charts Week #2 -- 20 Charts Week #3 -- 10 Charts Week #4 -- 22 Charts
2. Go through all charts identifying necessary or desired treatment. Complete tracking sheet.			
3. Contact all people by telephone. Try to schedule an appointment for treatment or for an exam and cleaning.	Patt	20 phone calls per week	Week #1 -- 20 contacts 8 appointments 4 Doctor -- 4 Hygiene Week #2 -- 15 contacts 4 appointments 2 Doctor -- 2 Hygiene Week #3 -- 21 contacts 6 appointments 2 Doctor 4 Hygiene Week #4 -- 18 contacts 5 appointments 3 Doctor 4 Hygiene
4.			
5.			(People were receptive to the financing program. Time was a barrier for many people. Should we consider extended hours?)
6.			

Figure 3–11 Writing the goal; designing the plan.

- Do they have dental insurance? If so, which plan? What is the coverage? Does it cover preventive care?

- How much dentistry has been diagnosed and left incomplete? (note the date of treatment plan to see if it is still current) (Fig. 3–12)

2. Once the data has been gathered for "this week's charts", make courteous marketing telephone calls to those patients to (1) express your concern about

KEY: HCFP= HEALTHCARE FINANCING PROGRAM

CHART AUDITS

DATE CONTACTED	PATIENT	PHONE	LAST DATE SEEN	AMOUNT OF DENTISTRY DIAGNOSED	INS.	HCFP	DATE APPLICATION SENT	DATE APPLICATION RECEIVED	COMMENTS
1. 2/23	Mary Jones	783-4421	12/5	$1000.00	$500.00	$35/mo.	2/24	3/7	Call to schedule when application is approved.
2. 2/23	Sam Murray	783-2209	11/1	$495.00	NO	$35/mo.	2/24	3/7	Not interested.
3. 2/23	Joel Coffey	226-4178	12/10	$1500.00	$750.00	$40/mo.	2/24	3/7	Scheduled appointment with hyg.
4. 2/23	Derrick Smith	783-7726	12/5		100%		2/24	3/7	Want to bring in rest of family when application approved. Call—
5.									
6.									
7.									
8.									
9.									
10.									
11.									
12.									
13.									
14.									

©Jameson Management Group, Inc.

Figure 3–12 Tracking device for chart audits

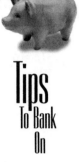

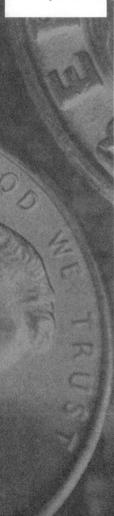

Tips To Bank On

You never know what you will get until you ask!

their care, (2) let them know you have not forgotten them, (3) reinforce the need for treatment, and (4) explain your new financing program. (Fig. 3–13)

Approach this effort steadily and with a positive attitude. Business tells us that 64% of the people promoting a service or a product never *ask*. You never know what you will get until you ask! The law of averages will work in your favor if you work on your entire set of charts.

Don't become discouraged if everyone doesn't jump at the idea. They won't. If you will get a positive response from 20-30 percent of the people contacted, you will have served your purpose well. Everyone will be a winner—you, the practice, and, most of all, the patient. At this time, you can introduce your healthcare financing program, so that you can clear the way for that patient to come in and say "Yes" to the dentistry.

To reiterate, then: First of all there needs to be a monitor created to track your work, your auditing efforts. Set a goal as to how many charts you will evaluate per week. How many charts do you feel that your practice can comfortably audit in a week's time? Make that decision. How many charts are you going to audit in a week? This is step one.

1. The team *sets the goal.*

2. The *objectives and strategies* of how the team is going to accomplish the goal of auditing the charts are defined. What are you going to do? How are you going to do it?

3. The *person or persons* responsible for each specific task are assigned their specifically detailed duties.

4. The *time frame* is set. Time activate each step.

5. *Evaluate.* You must be able to evaluate your progress and your success. Therefore, the monitor becomes critical, otherwise, how could you measure your progress?

Let me give you and example; Follow along with me on Fig. 3–12. Staff Y decides that they would do a chart audit of all of their charts. Let's say they had 2000 active charts in their

Telephone Campaign Script
Chart Audit

Business Manager: Good Morning, Mrs. Jones. This is Cathy from Dr. Jameson's office. Mrs. Jones, Dr. Jameson was reviewing your chart and noticed that at your last examination he had recommended treatment. (Here give a brief description of the recommended treatment stressing the end results and the benefits of the treatment.)

Mrs. Jones, at the same time that I am calling to reinforce the need for this treatment, I am also calling to tell you about a new financing program that we have available in our practice. It's called (Name of Company). (Name of Company) is a financing program for healthcare that allows people to finance their dentistry, and then to pay this out over a long period of time with the monthly payments being very comfortable.

We have found that many of our patients have found this program to be a convenient way to finance necessary and desired dental care.

Mrs. Jones, if you were to become involved with (Name of Company) and you financed the dentistry that Dr. Jameson has recommended to you, your first monthly payment would be approximately $50. It is a revolving plan which means that every time you make a payment, your next one is less.

Tell me, Mrs. Jones, would this be something that would be of interest to you?

Good. You could stop by the office to complete an application, or, if you prefer, I will mail an application to your home. Which would be best for you? Once we receive your application and when you are extended a line of credit, we will call to schedule an appointment to proceed with your treatment.

We believe that this is one of the best services we have been able to offer to our patients."

Figure 3–13 Telephone script for chart audits.

practice that they are going to audit. We will consider a patient who has been seen within the last two years an active patient. That's the *goal. The objectives and strategies* state they are going to start at chart X and are going through each of the charts *outlining* on the tracking sheets the date the person was contacted, the person's name, telephone number, if the patient has insurance or not, if the patient is a part of the healthcare financing program at this time or not, and the last time they were seen by dentist or hygienist. If the person is interested in becoming involved with the financing program, the date the application was sent is noted. The next column is the date the application is returned, and the last column is for comments.

So let's say that Jan, who, in this example is the clinical assistant, is going to be doing the actual auditing of the charts. Patt, the business administrator, is going to be making the telephone calls. Now, follow along with my example on figure 3–11. They are going to make every effort to audit 20 charts per week. They felt that this was a comfortable number for them. They are going to evaluate at their weekly staff meeting to show the staff the results of these audits. They will be evaluating (1) how many patients were they able to contact, (2) how many of these patients scheduled an appointment either with the dentist or with the hygienist, and (3) if patients were unwilling to schedule, what were the predominant reasons. Having this vital information gives a practice a wonderful opportunity to learn areas that might need improvement or extra attention.

The chart audit serves several purposes. (1) It allows the patient to know that you are trying to fulfill your responsibility of taking care of them. (2) It gives you a chance to encourage people to remain active with your practice. (3) It gives you the opportunity to let people know about the new financing program that you have available in your practice.

For example, you audit a chart and realize that this person has some necessary dentistry that has been diagnosed but remains incomplete. You would call this person after their chart has been audited and say,

"Ms. Jones? This is Cathy, from Dr. Jameson's office. How are you? Ms. Jones, Dr. Jameson has been reviewing your records and realized that the bridge that he had recommended for you has not been completed at this time and he was concerned. He asked that I call you to see if you had any questions about the treatment that he has prescribed. Ms. Jones, I see that you have dental insurance through Aetna and that is great. Dental insurance has been so helpful to so many of our patients. It serves as a wonderful supplement to their health care budget.

One of the reasons we're calling is to tell you about an exciting new program that we have available in our practice— a program that many of our patients have found to be a wonderful complement to their dental insurance. Ms. Jones, we have become involved with a financing program for dentistry. This program allows our patients to "finance" their dentistry and pay it out over a long period of time with very small monthly payments. This program lets you finance the dental care including the balance after insurance pays.

"In reviewing your record, I see that the fee for the bridge that Dr. Jameson is recommending for you is approximately $1500. We estimate your insurance company will pay about $750. Therefore, you would need to finance the balance or the other $750. If you become involved with our extended payment plan, you could go ahead and finance the balance that the insurance doesn't cover and your monthly payments would be approximately $35 a month. This is a revolving plan which means that every time you make a payment your next is less. Would this be something of interest to you?

Then she will say "yes" or "no" or she might have some other questions to ask you about the program. If she says "Oh yes, I would love this. I have wanted to have that bridge done. I am sick of the way my mouth is, and I would really like to have this done, but there was no way I could afford it. I didn't have $750 but I can pay $35 a month"; then you could say, "Ms. Jones, if you are going to be in our area I would encourage you to come by the office and pick up an application. If that is going to be a problem for you, I could drop one in the mail to you. Which would be best for you?" So she says, "Why don't you drop one of those in the mail to me."

Any time an application goes out of you office, track the date that the application is sent. Again, look at the tracking sheet. Note the date you sent the application, and as we discussed earlier, evaluate this chart audit at each staff meeting. The next column on the tracking sheet asks for the date that the application was received. If you notice that you sent Ms. Jones an application two weeks ago and you have not received the application back in the office, that is an alert. It is time to make a phone call to Ms. Jones. "Ms. Jones? This is Cathy from Dr. Jameson's office. I sent an application to your home regarding our extended payment plan and I haven't received that application back in the office. I wondered if you had received it. Oh, you have? Good. Do you have any questions or is there anything I can do to help?

"No? Then why don't you just drop that back in the mail and we will get it processed. Wonderful. I look forward to receiving the application. When I do receive the information, I will make sure that it is taken care of quickly. Once we find that you have been *extended* that credit line, I'll contact you and we will schedule an appointment to continue your treatment."

Because of your ongoing evaluations, you will always know when an application has left the office and if it has not been mailed back. The tracking devise or monitor lets you to know this. Otherwise you can see how a lot of information could fall through the cracks. Evaluation—or monitoring—is like taking the temperature of the practice. If you see that the temperature is rising (or if the monitors are indicating negative information) this is a symptom of a disease. This measurement gives you a chance to do something about it. If you don't track information about your practice, you lose the opportunity to correct any mistakes or problems. Track this chart audit and the mailing of your applications. Otherwise the applications will be floating around, and you won't have any idea where they are.

When you do reach a person—whether or not they wish to become involved with your financing program—you will want to either schedule the patients for treatment with the dentist or with the hygienist for continuous care. Most dentists feel that if the diagnosis has been made in the last six months that it is appropriate to schedule treatment with the dentist. However, if the patient has not been seen in the last six months, he/she needs to be scheduled for a periodic evaluation with the dentist as well as a professional cleaning with the hygienist.

Set a goal of having approximately 20% of the patients that you contact through the chart audit schedule an appointment, either with the dentist or the hygienist. This is a pretty realistic goal. Sometimes you will have a 50 or 60% acceptance rate. That is great. But if you receive a 20 to 30% acceptance rate, that is good. Don't be hard on yourself if you don't have a higher acceptance rate than that. Remember not to become discouraged if patients say no to your recommendation to schedule an appointment. First, you have fulfilled your responsibility to try and complete treatment. Second, you have let patients know that care about them, and third, you have introduced them to a wonderful new financial option that you have available in your practice. This might not mean anything to them today, but you are planting a seed for the future.

Don't try to audit all of the charts at once. Audit on a regular basis, consistently, and with a plan. Audit enough charts to fill one of the chart audit monitors, 14 patients per page. Then, get on the phone and make contact with those patients. Sometimes, offices avoid the telephone calls, so they audit all of the charts, fill lots of pages of information, but never get around to calling the people. Evaluate enough charts to fill one page, then call those people. Then go to another page and so on.

You are going to take many small steps and pretty soon you will have completed the long walk. What a fantastic way to expand your practice and to maximize this new financing program you have available in your practice.

INSURANCE

As you do your chart audit you may find that many people are putting off their dental treatment in spite of the fact that they have dental insurance. Available benefits are not being used, because these people may not be able to handle the balance after insurance pays.

Therefore, when you contact these people during your chart audit, let them know that you will file their insurance as a service to them. Tell them that if they choose to extend the payments on the balance after insurance pays, that you have a new, convenient way for them to *take care* of the balance. Then, tell them about your financing program.

On an ongoing basis, tell your insured patients about this opportunity, to utilize insurance benefits and to also have convenient monthly payments for the balance after insurance pays. You will find that more of your patients will use their insurance. Again, a win/win for everyone.

INSURANCE MANAGEMENT

Let's talk about insurance. The insurance program in your office is a system. It is a system that needs and deserves special attention because, as I said earlier, approximately 50% of the revenue of most dental practicies comes in the form of an insurance check. Whether you are computerized or not, there are certain criteria that must be in place in regard to insurance.

Gather relevant information about the benefit package from a patient's insurance plan. Necessary information to be gathered is as follows: (1) the employer, (2) the carrier, (3) the phone number, (4) the address, (5) the contact person, (6) the deductible, (7) maximum per year, and (8) the coverage types—preventive, basic, major, ortho, and other, and, of course, the information on the patient/policy holder.

Having this information will allow the business manager, when she makes financial arrangements, to make a close estimate of the expected insurance portion and the private pay portion on which she will need to make financial arrangements. If that private pay portion after insurance pays is a barrier to acceptance of treatment, you can finance it with your payment plan.

Many people have dental insurance but do not take advantage of their yearly maximum because they cannot afford the difference that insurance does not cover. When you are performing your chart audit, you may find, to your amazement, that people have necessary or desired dental treatment, and they have dental insurance. However, the treatment is sitting in the charts waiting to be done. What's preventing the person from going ahead? Probably money.

I have even seen cases in which patients receive a predetermination of benefits from an insurance company but are not able to schedule an appointment because they can't afford the balance after the insurance pays. I introduce them to our financing program, and they are able to say "yes" to the treatment.

We need to phase people's treatment from time to time. We make careful record of the necessary treatment, the phases that have been completed, and the phases that are yet to be completed. We know the total investment, the expected insurance coverage, and the personal responsibility on the part of the patient. If the patient must spread the treatment over a period of time in order to receive the care, we will utilize yearly maximums in conjunction with their available credit on their financing program. We would rather phase the treatment than compromise the care. Of course, the dentist would phase the treatment only if it were beneficial to the patient.

Please be insurance aware. In other words, do all you can do to help a person maximize his/her insurance benefits. But do not become insurance driven which means, do not let what an insurance company will or will not cover determine the type of treatment you recommend. Remember, insurance companies are not interested in whether or not the treatment you are recommending is best for the patient. They are interested in whether or not it is a covered benefit and will pay accordingly.

One other helpful service now being offered by financing companies and bank cards is pre-authorization forms that can be completed by the patients and kept in their charts. (Fig. 1–1) With these pre-authorizations, the patient gives you permission to place any balances left on their financial program after insurance pays. You can also gain the patient's permission to place regular payments on the program if they are on a regular program of therapy or treatment.

Make it easy for people to pay, convenience is important to busy people in today's world. Insurance has been a wonderful supplement to people's dental care and to the growth of dental practices. Now more people can use insurance benefits because they have a way to finance the difference after insurance pays.

Tips
To Bank
On

. . . be insurance aware . . . . But do not become insurance driven . . .

FACTS REGARDING
DENTAL INSURANCE

(This has been around longer than me. I don't know who originally wrote this—but it's great!)

Dental insurance is rapidly playing a larger role in helping people obtain dental treatment. Since we strongly feel our patients deserve the best possible dental care we can provide, and in an effort to maintain this high quality care, we would like to share some facts about dental insurance with you.

Fact #1: Dental insurance is not meant to be a *pay-all*. It is only meant to be a supplement.

Fact #2: Many plans tell their insured that they'll be covered "up to 80% or up to 100%". In spite of what you're told, we've found most plans cover less than the average fee. Some plans pay more, some less. The amount your plan pays is determined by how much your employer paid for the plan. The less he paid for the insurance, the less you'll receive.

Fact #3: It has been the experience of many dentists that some insurance companies tell their customers that "fees are above the usual and customary fees" rather than saying to them that "our benefits are low". Remember, you get back only what your employer puts in, less the profits and administrative costs of the insurance company.

Fact #4: Many *routine* dental services are *not* covered by insurance plans.

Please do not hesitate to ask us any questions about our office policies. We want you to be comfortable in dealing with these matters, and we urge you to consult us if you have any questions regarding our services and/or fees. We will fill out and file insurance forms at no charge. We will do all we can to assure you of maximum benefits.

If we take assignment on your insurance, we feel that 60 days is a reasonable length of time for us to wait for payment from your insurance company.

Thank You!

INSURANCE OBJECTIONS

Patients must want the dentistry before the fee is presented. If they want the dentistry badly enough, the fee and the insurance will not be quite so overwhelming. However, when insurance objections do arise, the following verbal skills may prove beneficial:

Here are some normal objections/questions about dental insurance and appropriate responses.

1. *Does my insurance cover this? If it doesn't, I'm not sure I want to get this done!*

    "Ms. Jones, we'll do the best we can to maximize your insurance benefits. Then, we will work with you to find a way for you to handle the balance.

    Let me ask you this, if we can find a way to handle the financial aspect of your treatment, is this the type of dentistry you would like to receive."

    "Yes. But, I don't think I can afford it if my insurance doesn't cover it."

    "How much could you afford to invest per month?"

    "Oh, I could pay maybe $30 or $40 per month, but no more."

    "Let me tell you this. With the information we have from your insurance company, we estimate that they will cover approximately $1000. That's your yearly maximum. That would leave a balance of $500. We will establish a line of credit for you with our healthcare financing program and for less than $30 per month, you can go ahead with the treatment that the doctor has recommended. Does that work for you?"

    "Yes. That would be fine."

2. *If my insurance doesn't cover this, why do you say that I need it?*

"Dental insurance is a supplement to your healthcare. It is not a payall. The benefits that are available to you are based on the amount your employer paid for the policy. The less he pays—the less your receive. Predefined benefits have nothing to do with necessary treatment."

3. *My insurance covers 100% of my dental care. My employer said it did.*

"Many insurance programs say that they will pay 100% or 80% . What they don't say that this is a percentage of their fees—not ours."

4. *My insurance company says that your fees are above the usual and customary! Why are your fees above average?*

"Our fees reflect our commitment to quality. Insurance companies provide a great service by supplementing your healthcare, but their benefits are not determined by the quality of the care, only on the amount of premium."

5. *This costs too much.*

"Today, most things do. Tell me, how much too much is it?"

6. *I have to think this over.*

"Ms. Jones, I know you wouldn't take the time to think this over if you weren't seriously interested. Tell me what is it that you need to think over, the dentistry itself, whether Dr. Jameson will do the dentistry, or the financial aspect of the dentistry?"

7. *I can't believe I need this much. How in the world did this happen?*

"I understand your concern. Many factors have affected your oral health . We can't change what's happened up to now, but we can change the situation that exists and restore your mouth to health again. Then, let's mutually commit to keeping it healthy. You'll make an investment now and then we'll work together to insure that investment with an excellent program of maintenance and home care."

MORE ABOUT INSURANCE MANAGEMENT

As I have said, for most dental practices, 50% of the income comes in the form of an insurance check. In other words approximately one half of the collections of the practice comes from insurance. Thus, it is imperative that the insurance aspect of the practice be managed and monitored with extreme dedication.

Management systems in the dental practice need to be both time-efficient and cost-efficient. The insurance management system is no exception. Insurance has been, and will remain, an asset to dental practices. The following graph illustrates the percentage of people who have dental insurance. (Fig. 3–14)

And so, obviously, if this many patients have dental insurance and this much of dental practice income comes from dental insurance, a devoted concentration on the filing and follow-up

Who Has Dental Insurance?

- 60% of the population has dental insurance
- 73% of their dental bill is paid by insurance
- Population having dental insurance by income

UNDER $30,000	$30,000—$45,000	OVER $45,000
37%	62%	70%

*adjusted for inflation to 1996 levels

Source: Dr. T. Warren Center

Figure 3–14

Tips To Bank On

Keeping up in a regular, systematic manner prevents insurance overload; loss of control, and slow cash flow from insurance.

of insurance is essential. The following is a simple, yet effective, way to manage your insurance on a daily basis. Keeping up in a regular, systematic manner prevents insurance *overload;* loss of control, and slow cash flow from insurance.

Suggested Procedure:

Step 1: File insurance daily. The most expedient and acceptable manner to file insurance (if you are not computerized) is to attach a copy of your superbill, with the day's completed treatments, to the patient's insurance form. (The only insurance form that should be kept in a patient's file is the original insurance form with the top filled out and the assignment of benefits section signed. Then you will be able to copy this claim for future use.)

Note: Even if you are computerized, the following method of filing and follow-up is appropriate:

Step 2: Mail this original superbill and insurance claim or ADA claim off the computer to the appropriate insurance company. Make sure that necessary X-rays are included in those cases that require X-ray. Also include a narrative that describes a particular situation, if a description would expedite the processing of the claim. Sending these with the original claim will minimize refiling slow-downs.

Step 3: Develop a set of files—January through December. Then, on a daily basis, file a copy of the insurance claim along with a copy of the superbill—where used—into the appropriate month. When you do this on a daily basis, you will acquire an automatic chronological filing of insurance claims.

Step 4: Develop another set of files January through December for predetermination of benefits. The predetermination of benefits are to be filed in the same manner as the claims for services rendered. These need to be filed in a separate set of files, however, for appropriate tracking of this necessary dentistry.

Step 5: On a daily basis, go to your January through December files to see if any claims or predetermination of benefits are 30 days past due. Your chronological filing system will provide you with a quick analysis of this information.

Step 6: Develop another set of files, A–Z. When a claim is paid and you receive an Explanation of Benefits, or an EOB, go to your January through December file and pull the appropriate claim. Check to make sure that you have received the correct payment for the services rendered. Then, attach the EOB to the claim and file this under the patient's name. In other words, file these paid claims alphabetically. This allows for quick access to a patient's claim if questions should arise. At the end of a year, pull the paid claims and file them away in a storage area. (The length of time that you need to keep these paid claims varies from state to state. Contact your state insurance commissioner and find out how long you are required to keep these paid claims). Then your A–Z files are ready to receive the paid claims for the new year.

Step 7: Check your January through December files on a daily basis. When a claim is 30 days past due, call the particular insurance company to see what the problem might be. If they indicate that they "never received the claim" or if "something is missing and you need to refile", do so *that day!* Make a copy of the previously filed claim and refile. At the top of the second copy, write *refiled* (or *second filing*) and the date. Then put your copy back in the original filing location. You want to know the exact amount of time that has passed since the original filing.

The following information must be gathered for each insurance company with which you work. (Fig. 3–15)

This insurance information allows you (1) to make excellent financial arrangements and (2) to make appropriate calls when there is a question about a particular claim.

Calling the insurance companies when a claim is past due or when there is a question about a claim will expedite the receiving of the payment. If there is a question about a claim, timely telephone follow-up will let you know where you stand— and if, in fact, a refiling does need to take place.

Insurance management is a very involved, vital job responsibility. The responsibility needs to be given to a specific person on the business office. The details of how the responsibility is to be handled need to be outlined, and intricate training needs to take place. Time for the management of the insurance aspect of the practice needs to be allocated and prioritized. Realizing that approximately 50% of the practice's income is derived from insurance validates this time and responsibility allotment.

If you are not presently computerized and are not doing electronic claims filing—do so ! Immediately. Turnaround of money is usually within seven to ten working days. There are fewer lost claims and fewer requests for X-rays and for back-up data. Filing is as simple as making a telephone call to initiate your modem. Follow-up is still necessary but will be much less time consuming.

CONTINUOUS CARE

Many people do not stay on a regular program of continuous care of hygiene, or they do not involve all members of their family in your program, because the total investment per visit is prohibitive. That's the last thing any of you want— for your patients to put off needed or desired care because of the "cost".

Introducing the financing program through the hygienists and through your hygiene retention program will not only allow more of your patients to receive this valuable service, but it will

Insurance Information

EMPLOYER: _____

CARRIER: _____

TELEPHONE: _____

ADDRESS: _____

_____

CONTACT PERSON: _____

ANNUAL MAXIMUM : _____ DEDUCTIBLE: _____

COVERAGE TYPES: _____

PREVENTIVE: _____ BASIC: _____

MAJOR: _____ ORTHO: _____

OTHER: _____

COMMENTS: _____

_____

_____

_____

_____

Figure 3–15

also help you to further develop this *lifeblood* of the dental practice.

If you are involved with a non-surgical periodontal program, or if you are offering sealant therapy, you know that many patients want and need this care but find the financial responsibility difficult. However, if they find that they can obtain quality preventive care for themselves and their families and that the monthly investment will fit nicely into the family budget, many will proceed. (Fig. 3–16)

CASE PRESENTATION

At the time of your case presentation or consultation appointment, introduce the financing program to your clients/patients. Otherwise, as you are trying to educate the patient about the services you are offering, they may be thinking of nothing but the *cost*. The human mind can only think of one thing at a time. Therefore, if a patient is calculating what they think the treatment will cost, they may not hear a word you are saying.

If you think something may be a barrier to acceptance, it is better to address this potential barrier before the patient brings it up. In this manner you have a chance to turn a potential negative into a positive.

Example:

You might say something like this:

> "Ms. Jones, before I tell you what I have diagnosed and before I explain the treatment that I believe will help us obtain excellent oral health for you, let me first tell you that if you have any concern about the financing of the dentistry that we have convenient financial options right here in our practice. Before we proceed with treatment, we will make sure that you are comfortable with the financing of the treatment.
>
> But for right now, if you agree, I would like to discuss the treatment I feel would be best for you. Let's focus on those recommendations and then we will discuss the financing thoroughly. Does that sound good to you?"

Then, once she has agreed, proceed with your presentation. You will get a lot more accomplished in a much shorter period of time. There will be fewer misunderstandings. Greater acceptance of your treatment plans will result.

Offer the best treatment possible, make the financing of the dentistry comfortable, and then get out of the way. Let the patient make the decision of whether or not to proceed. (Figs. 3–17 and 3–18)

Dear _____:

This is just a short reminder that you have not been in for your appointment concerning your dental hygiene care and evaluation. We have attempted to schedule this appointment for some time now with no success.

The purpose of this appointment is to prevent the formation or development of any gross dental problems. One problem that can occur is periodontal (or gum) disease. Loss of teeth due to bone degeneration can happen quickly and quietly and can go unnoticed without regular dental care.

Please don't ignore this notice! It is very important to maintain great oral health by visiting our office on a regular basis.

Sincerely,

Special Note: Remember to ask about our new financing program. Finance your dentistry for a small amount each month. No more reason to put off valuable care for you and your family because of cost.

Figure 3–16 Hygiene retention letter

OVERCOMING OBJECTIONS TO YOUR FINANCING PROGRAM

THE PRESENTATION

The presentation of a healthcare financing program makes all the difference in the world. The program will work in direct proportion to your belief in the program as an asset to your practice and to your patients and in direct proportion to your

Tips To Bank On

Offer the best treatment possible, make the financing of the dentistry comfortable, and then get out of the way.

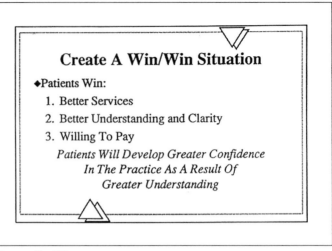

Figure 3–17

ability to present and market the program. How you communicate these programs will make them work or will leave you with little success. *Great Communication = Great Production.* (Who said that?)

You will need to spend time, as a team, going over these communication skills so that everyone is comfortable with them. When patients ask questions, everyone on the team can answer those questions enthusiastically and competently. The more excited you are about this new financing program, the more excited your patients will be and the more receptive they will be to your suggestions. The patients will be a reflection of you. Your success will be in direct proportion to your enthusiasm.

How to Present
a Healthcare Financing Program

Pay close attention to the following presentation script. Notice, in fact, count the number of benefits I stress to the patient. A person's behavior will be driven by "what's in this for

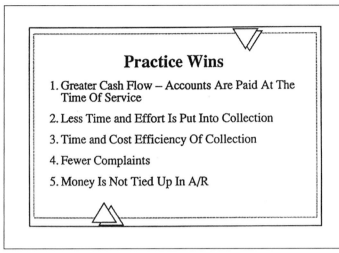

Practice Wins

1. Greater Cash Flow – Accounts Are Paid At The Time Of Service

2. Less Time and Effort Is Put Into Collection

3. Time and Cost Efficiency Of Collection

4. Fewer Complaints

5. Money Is Not Tied Up In A/R

Figure 3–18

me". If you intend for a person to accept your offer to become involved with a financing program, you must present the program in terms of how that program will benefit the patient. Memorize this script. Practice it with each other. Then, present the program to the patient in exactly this way. Of course, you will individualize the verbal skills to fit you. However, "if it ain't broke, don't fix it." These verbal skills have worked for thousands of people—hundreds of practices. I would give it a try if I were you.

"Ms. Jones, I am glad to tell you that we do have a wonderful method of long term financing right here in our practice. The program is called, ABC Financing Program. ABC is a financing program for healthcare only—dentistry in our case. You apply right here in our office. The application is very easy to complete and will take only a few minutes. We will send your application to the company for processing and once you have received a line of credit, we can provide your dental treatment, finance the treatment with ABC

Company, and spread the payments out over a long period of time thus making your payments very small—payments that will fit nicely into your monthly budget.

Dr. Jameson has paid all necessary fees for you to become involved with the company and there is no yearly fee. It works kind of like dental insurance, except that you will only pay for the service when you use it.

Ms. Jones, based on the treatment that Dr. Jameson is recommending for you, your first monthly payment would be approximately $30. It is a revolving payment program which means that every time you make a payment your next one is less. In other words, for about $30 per month, you can receive the very best treatment we can provide.

Does this sound like something that would be of interest to you? "

At the same time that you are learning to present the program, you will want to learn how to defuse negatives that might come up during the presentation. You will want to defuse the negatives associated with this new payment option, and you will want to build a patient's confidence in the fact that the program will help them. Patients must understand the benefits of the program, or they will not accept.

Here are some common situations you will probably encounter and suggested verbal skills for addressing these situations.

Example: You have been practicing dentistry for a while and your patients have been paying you small monthly payments for ever—and ever—and ever.

Business Administrator: "Ms. Jones let me tell you about a new program we have in our office. We have found that many of our patients need long-term comfortable financing to handle their dental care. We now have available in our practice a method of long-term financing called ABC Financing Company.

This company has joined our team as our financial partner.

Ms. Jones, you can apply for the financing program right here in our practice. You don't have to go anywhere. Once you are extended a line of credit, we can finance your dentistry and you can pay it out over a long period of time and your payments will be very small."

Ms. Jones: "What are you talking about? I have been paying Dr. Jameson forever? Why can't I just keep paying him out the way I always have?"

Business Administrator: "We are still offering long term payment plans. We are just doing it in a better way. We have been advised by our accountant that it is neither time nor cost efficient to run a banking business within our practice. We decided it was better for our patients if we concentrated on what we do best and that is providing excellent dental care.

We have become associated with a reputable company that offers long term extended payments to our patients. This company works with us to offer this convenient financing. In addition, Ms. Jones, we are committed to maintaining comfortable fees for our dental services, and so we have searched for a better, more cost efficient way to offer long term payments."

Ms. Jones: "Well, what is this program? Please explain this to me."

Business Administrator: "It is a financing company that features an extended payment plan for healthcare only. By having a line of credit established for your healthcare, you can conveniently budget this vital service into your monthly income."

Ms. Jones: "I don't know about this. Is it hard to apply or to get accepted?"

Business Administrator: "You asked a good question, Ms. Jones, and I am glad to tell you that the application is quite easy and the acceptance rate is

81

quite high. In fact you apply right here in our office. The application will be similar to any application you have filled out previously. However, if you do have any questions, I'll be more than happy to help you."

Ms. Jones: "Well, are they going to charge me interest?"

Business Administrator: "There is a service fee, Ms. Jones, just as you pay with any other financing program. The service fee is 1.625 % a month or about $1.63 per month for every $100 that you finance, and Ms. Jones that is not much considering the fact that you can receive the treatment that the doctor has recommended to you and not have to make a major investment all at once."

Ms. Jones: "Well I don't know about this. I just wish I could pay Dr. Jameson the way I used to."

Business Administrator: "I know how you feel. We have other good, long term patients that felt confused about the changes we are making until they found out that they could still spread out the payments for their dental care. However, heir monthly payments are usually smaller and they can take longer to pay out their balance. Ms. Jones we have many families using this program and they just love the convenience. These families seem to be happier because with their available line of credit they are better able to take care of more members of their family on a more regular basis."

Ms. Jones: "Well how much will my monthly payments be?"

Business Administrator: "You are only required to pay 3% of the existing balance. Dr. Jameson has recommended treatment for you that places your responsibility at $1000. Your first monthly payment will be approximately $30. It is a revolving program which means that every time you make a payment the next payment will be less. Would that be comfortable for you?"

Of course you would have to supplement the percentages, service fee rates and monthly rates according to your own program. But study these verbal skills and scripts. Put these skills into your own words and become comfortable with them. The presentation of the program is three-fourths of it.

Again, everyone on the team must have confidence in the program, and know how to present the program and address and overcome objections.

Once your financial system is in place in the practice, everyone on the team must provide support for the program. It is very difficult for a business manager to make financial arrangements with the patients based on the financial policy only to have exceptions made on a regular basis.

I am not suggesting that the dentist does not have the option to make an exception to a policy. He/she should certainly have that option. However, the business manager must know that she will be supported and *backed up* by the dentist and the entire team.

If a patient asks a question about financing or money or cost in the clinical area, here is how I recommend you handle those kinds of questions.

Example:

> **Patient:** "The doctor says I need a crown. How much is that? And, how can I pay for that ?"
>
> **Dr./Clinical Assistant/or Hygienist:** "Ms. Jones, are you concerned about the financing of your crown? Will that make a difference as to whether or not you go ahead with treatment?"
>
> **Patient:** "Well, yes."
>
> **Dr./Clinical Assistant/ or Hygienist:** "Ms. Jones, we have several generous financial options for our patients. Jan, our business administrator handles all financial arrangements, and she is terrific. I will let her know that you are concerned about the financing of your crown. She will tell you the total investment and the options

we have available for payment. I am sure that she will be able to work something out for you."

In the above dialogue, the clinical team did not close the door on the financial question. They left the door open for the patient and for the business administrator. They gave a very positive introduction to the financial options and they gave a professional compliment to the business administrator. A compliment of this kind from the clinical team can make the financial discussion go much smoother.

Clinical team, you must be careful not to close the door to a positive financial discussion and you must not give the patient the idea that a discussion of money is a taboo thing or that the fees are so high that you wouldn't want to touch such a discussion with a ten foot pole.

Your confidence will give the financial coordinator/business administrator a smoother path. Get the above verbal skills down pat and use them whenever you are asked a financial/money question in the clinical area.

A TEAM EFFORT

The team needs to spend time going over all of this financial information—the defining of the policy, the integration of a financing program into the practice, the verbal skills of presenting the program and of overcoming objections. A strategic plan of action for the marketing of the financing program needs to be determined, written, and implemented.

By becoming involved with and by maximizing a healthcare financing program, not only do *you* win by running a more cost-effective credit business, but *your patients* win, because they are able to have the care that they want and need. One more benefit is that dentists are able to do the dentistry they were taught to do in dental school. Making the financing of the dentistry comfortable for the patient by defusing the *fear of cost* makes it possible for people to receive quality, optimum, complete dentistry rather than partial or incomplete dentistry or *patchwork dentistry.*

Gather information about these financial programs and study this information together as a team. Decide which one will work best for you. Which one can you get behind and get excited about and really support? Which one do you think will help build your practice and serve your patients best? This financial system offers firmness while at the same time offers incredible flexibility.

Tips
To Bank On

This financial system offers firmness while at the same time offers incredible flexibility.

Making Financial Arrangements: Getting Ready

*"It isn't only what you do,
or even how you do it—
but also when you do it."*

— MARK MCCORMACK
THE 110% SOLUTION

Now you have a financial policy in your practice. You have become involved with a healthcare financing program. You have put a dam in the river called "accounts receivable" and you are no longer carrying long term accounts on your own books. You have spent time, as a team, discussing and developing the financial system in your practice. You are ready to go.

In order to be effective in making a financial arrangement with a patient, you have to start with the right mind set. You must be totally committed to the belief that the patient needs the dental care, and that he/she will benefit tremendously from your services. Everyone on the team must believe that if a patient

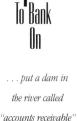

**Tips
To Bank
On**

*. . . put a dam in
the river called
"accounts receivable"*

Tips
To Bank
On

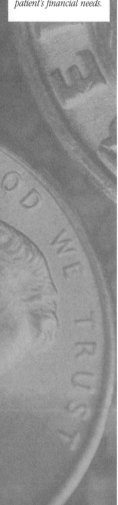

Your job, then, will be to find a solution to every patient's financial needs.

walks out the door not scheduling an appointment—that the patient loses just as much as you do, or more.

If your attitude is in the right place and you have this type of commitment, then you will see the making of the financial arrangement as a challenge—a challenge to determine each patient's financial situation and their concerns, if any. Your job, then, will be to find a *solution* to every patient's financial needs. (Fig. 4–1)

To be effective with your financial arrangements, you need the following:

(1) Privacy: Remember, the oral cavity is an intimate zone of a person's body and so is the pocketbook. Therefore, you need to be in a quiet area that provides the necessary privacy. Do not try to make a financial arrangement at the front desk in front of everyone in the office—team members and other patients.

When financial arrangements are "attempted" at the front desk, several negative things can happen.

> (a) A person may become embarrassed and may schedule the appointment but have no intention to come to the appointment. He/she may not feel comfortable telling

---

To Lead a Person To a Buying Decision, One Must Have:

1. Knowledge Of Product Or Service

2. In Depth Knowledge Of Money And Financing

3. Ability To Complete Any Necessary Paperwork

Figure 4–1

you that they have a concern about the fee and he/she may not want to ask you for financial options for fear that other people will overhear the conversation.

(b) The business administrator may be interrupted by people checking in, or by the telephone, or by another person coming to the front desk to check out. If there are interruptions during the conversation regarding the fee, mistakes can be made easily. Attention cannot be focused on the person with whom she is making the arrangement. Or, if there are too many interruptions and the conversation becomes impossible, there may be no financial arrangement made whatsoever. This, of course, can lead to poor collections and, sometimes, disgruntled patients who were not informed of their financial responsibility in advance.

And so, for all reasons, make your financial arrangements in private. If you do not have a formal consultation area, find some place in the office where a small but neat area can be prepared for the consultations, like the dentist's private office.

Personal Note:

In our office, we removed an unnecessary couch from John's private office and put a table with three chairs in its place. On that table is the view box for necessary radiographs and in the drawer is the necessary paperwork. An intra-oral camera is in the consultation area, as well as a computer terminal networked with our management software.

John makes his presentation of recommendations, with his business administrator/treatment coordinator/financial coordinator present. Once he has completed his presentation and is sure that the patient has no further clinical questions for him, he turns the consultation over to the financial coordinator and excuses himself.

The financial coordinator has heard everything he has said to the patient. In fact, she discussed the treatment plan with him before the consultation appointment so that she would know what he wanted to do, why and how he wanted to proceed—

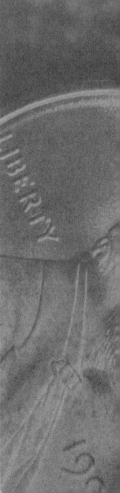

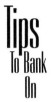

Tips To Bank On

. . . make your financial arrangements in private.

what he wants to do first, second, and so on, and how long he needs for each appointment. (Fig. 4–2)

She is fully prepared to give the doctor *quality* third party reinforcement. She will be able to answer possible clinical questions that the patient may not have been comfortable asking the doctor. (The person presenting the financial consultation needs to have clinical knowledge so that she can give this type of backup and so that she can answer—in layman's language—questions that *will* come up during her time with the patient.)

Once the doctor has excused him/herself, the financial coordinator takes over. She needs to ask the following question before the discussion of finances begins:

"Ms. Jones, I know that Dr. Jameson asked if you had any questions and you said no, but I thought there might be something you would like to ask me."

Again, the reason for this critical question is that the clinical questions must be answered before a person will go ahead. Clear any questions about the procedures/treatment, the course of action to be taken, and give statements related to the benefits of the treatment. Sell the person on the treatment first—then discuss the fee.

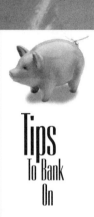

Tips To Bank On

Sell the person on the treatment first—then discuss the fee.

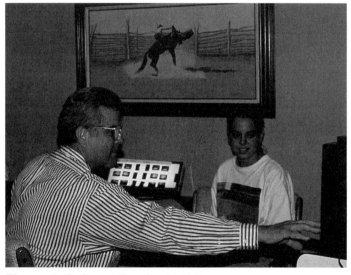

Figure 4–2 Presenting the dentistry.

Do not be in a rush. Have time to answer questions and discuss any concerns. Know that the discussion with the financial coordinator might be longer than the discussion with the dentist about the treatment. That's OK. This is a person who wants or needs your care. Your responsibility is to make a financial arrangement that will allow him/her to go ahead. You want a clear, written financial arrangement before the discussion is complete and you will want to have scheduled at least the first appointment.

Trying to close too fast may be worse than not trying to close at all.

If you are in an office where there is a small number of team persons and only one person in the business office, you can still do this. Pre-block your appointment book for the dentist's consultation time and the financial coordinator's time. Knowing in advance that the business administrator will be occupied with a patient discussing finances makes it possible for her to "get covered". The clinical assistant can check people in and out during that time. Put a bell or chime on your front door so that she will hear when a patient arrives and, if need be, place a special message on your telephone so that you can gather necessary data from incoming calls and can return the calls immediately.

If you have more than one clinical assistant, she can answer the telephone. What you don't want is for the financial coordinator to be interrupted to handle front desk responsibilities or to answer the telephone while she is having a private financial arrangement conversation with a patient. That's a great way to lose the patient and to lose the case.

(2) Professional Image: The business administrator/financial coordinator needs to be dressed in business attire presenting a very professional image. She is going to be making a financial/business arrangement with the patient. She has a totally different relationship with the patient than does the clinical team. Sitting down with a person talking about the financial responsibility for his/her dental care needs to be done in a business-like atmosphere. That includes the atmosphere or aura created by the person making that arrangement.

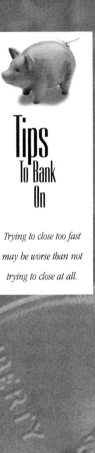

Tips To Bank On

Trying to close too fast may be worse than not trying to close at all.

(3) Introductions: In most instances, the patient will already know the person who is going to be making the financial arrangement. The patient would have met her on the telephone and in the business office. Or, if a member of your clinical team is serving the role of treatment coordinator, the patient may have met her during the initial comprehensive evaluation appointment.

However, if you are in a large office where a person is handling all of the financial aspects of the practice, including the making of the financial arrangements, make sure that appropriate introductions are made.

"Ms. Jones, this is Jan Davis, my business administrator. I have asked her to join us today for our consultation. Jan will be working with you to make the financial arrangement and she will be helping with the scheduling of your appointments. I felt that it was very important that she hear what I am recommending for you. Is this all right with you?" (No one in our own practice has ever said "no" to that question.")

Note that the dentist not only introduced Jan, but he also told Ms. Jones what her role was in the consultation. He also stressed how much he wanted to make sure she knew exactly where they would be going with the treatment.

(4) Body Language: Watch for Buying Signs: All of the above mentioned reasons for having the financial coordinator join you for the consultation are excellent ones. However, one more significant reason is that she can watch the patient's body language for visual buying signs, or signs of discomfort. She can also hear the exchange between the doctor and the patient and will know what part of the treatment plan she may need to revisit. In addition, the patient will not be able to say, "Oh, no, the doctor said I could do this—or that". If she is sitting in the room, she will know exactly what the doctor did or did not say.

The financial/treatment coordinator needs to be *out of the way* and non-invasive during the doctors' discussion. She does not want to interfere in any way during the consultation. However, she does need to make notes that she will refer to during her time with the patient.

(5) Call the Patient by Name—Frequently: During your financial discussion, refer to the patient by name from time to time. The sweetest sound to a person's ear is the sound of his/her own name. Plus, a patient will feel that your time with him/her is more personalized. This bit of quality customer service is appropriate throughout the office by all members of the team but is critical during the intimate discussion of money.

(6) Have All Necessary Information: Be prepared. All of the appropriate information needs to be complete and in the consultation room during the financial consultation. The financial coordinator will have had the treatment plan in hand prior to the consultation so that she can calculate the fees, including the expected insurance coverage, if appropriate. She also needs to know what the first monthly payment would be the patient places the total fee—or the fee after insurance pays—with the healthcare financing program. (Fig. 4–3)

If a patient expresses a concern about money at his/her initial appointment, then have him/her complete an application for your financing program while in the office. Then, when he/she comes back for the consultation, you will already know if they have been extended a line of credit—or not—and how much that line of credit will be. This may prove to be valuable while you are making the arrangement.

You want to be so well prepared for this appointment that you do not have to figure information while the patient waits for you. You want to be so well prepared that you have all the necessary information to make just about any kind of financial arrangement. You want to have your "ducks in a row". Being well prepared says, "We want to take care of you—physically and financially". Being prepared says that you are professionals and handle all aspects of your relationship with a patient in a professional manner. (Fig. 4–4, 4–5)

Know that patients make decisions about your quality of care by everything, including how you handle their business relationship. You must be prepared in order to give excellent, *state of the art care.*

FINANCIAL AGREEMENT

YOUR DENTAL INSURANCE IS YOUR RESPONSIBILITY ... BUT **WE CAN HELP** ...
Regardless of what we might calculate as your dental benefit in dollars, we must stress the
fact that you, the patient, are responsible for the TOTAL TREATMENT FEE. As a courtesy
to you, we do accept assignment of benefit payments from most insurance companies.
This will reduce your immediate, out-of-pocket expenditures. The outlined estimate is based on
limited information obtained from your insurance company. We allow 60 days for your insurance
company to make payment. AFTER THIS TIME, ALL INQUIRIES (FOLLOW-UP) ON
PAYMENTS DUE BECOME YOUR RESPONSIBILITY.

DATE:_____ DEDUCTIBLE:_____ MAXIMUM BENEFIT PER YEAR:_____

PATIENT'S NAME:_____ SS# OF INSURED:_____

INSURED'S NAME:_____ EMPLOYER:_____

TOOTH NUMBER/S	RECOMMENDED TREATMENT	FEE	INSURANCE PMT. EST.	PATIENT PMT. EST.
	TOTAL			

Payment Option Accepted

Financial Agreement

I accept the TREATMENT PLAN above:_____ Date:_____
I agree to the FINANCIAL RESPONSIBILITY for the total fee. The fees listed on this
treatment outline will be honored for 90 days from the above date. After this time, the fees are
subject to adjustment.
REMARKS:_____

©Jameson Management Group, Inc.

Figure 4–3 Written financial agreement

SUMMARY

Have a team meeting to determine the who, what, how, when, why, and where of your financial arrangements. Make sure that you incorporate all the above six criteria in your discussion and in your protocol. Get your paperwork in order. Make sure that you have the location arranged and that it is conducive to a professionally presented financial discussion.

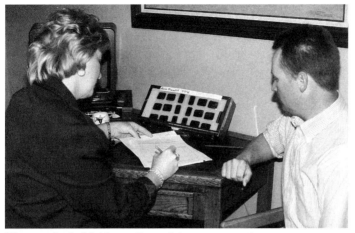

Figure 4–4 Making a financial arrangement.

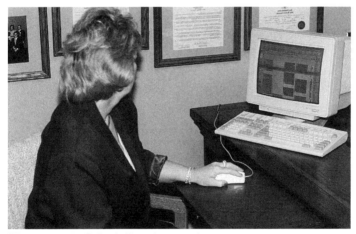

Figure 4–5 Scheduling the appointment

The person making the financial arrangements will be making the final close of the presentation. She has a critical responsibility. If a patient sees the benefits of treatment as presented by the dentist, then the only thing that may prevent him/her from going ahead will be the financing. Have everything work toward the goal of gaining a high rate of case acceptance, including financial acceptance.

Making Financial Arrangements: Communication And Verbal Skills

*"Communication skill is
the bottom line to your success."*

— C A T H Y   J A M E S O N ,   M . A .
*G R E A T   C O M M U N I C A T I O N =
G R E A T   P R O D U C T I O N*

T he environment has been prepared, the appropriate paperwork has been made available, the format of the financial presentation has been determined. Now, you are ready to prepare for the face-to-face presentation. In *Great Communication = Great Production,* I said that "communication skill is the bottom line to your success". Certainly, in the area of making financial arrangements, how you communicate with a patient will make or break the situation.

People   want you to help them find a solution to their financial situation, no matter what that may be. You must be a good listener. You must be able to peel the layers of the problem to determine the core or center of the problem. Then—and only

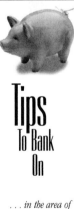

*. . . in the area of
making financial
arrangements, how you
communicate with a
patient will make or
break the situation.*

then—can you come to a cooperative decision as to how to solve that problem. (Fig. 5–1)

Communication:
The Bottom Line To Your Success

Presentation Skills

1. Ask Questions to Better Understand the Situation

2. Overcome Objections to Motivate the Patient to Pay

3. Offer Options to Gain a Commitment

Figure 5–1

" A problem is only a problem until it becomes defined. Once it becomes defined, it becomes manageable."

— MICHAEL DOYLE
HOW TO MAKE MEETINGS WORK

There's your challenge. Define the problem. Consider it a challenge—one that can be solved.

BUILDING A RELATIONSHIP OF TRUST AND CONFIDENCE

Establish a relationship with the patient before making financial arrangements, or in fact, before making a case presentation. Business experts tell us that people will never buy your product or service unless they have a strong relationship of trust and/or confidence with you. Without question, if people are going to invest in your services, they must have that trust. After all, you are going to be "in their mouth"—that intimate zone. Plus, you are going to be helping the patient to get healthy again—or you are going to be changing their smile.

Therefore, from the minute the telephone is answered, to the mailing of the welcome packet, to the initial appointment, to the making of the financial arrangements, and through the completion of treatment, each person on the team has what business calls a "moment of truth". Each person on the team has a chance to make or break a relationship with a patient. Each step of the patient's path must be based on the establishment and the continuation of trust.

If too many people are saying "I'd like to think it over", there is a problem in your system of personal/patient relationships.

When a person comes to you as a personal referral, that person will already have a certain level of trust and confidence. However, once they decide to come to the office, your people skills take over.

If you analyze your case acceptance ratio and are displeased with the level of acceptance, you may find—if you honestly evaluate each and every patient experience—that a trust level is not established before the financial responsibility is discussed. There is no reason to talk about money if the patient doesn't see the benefit of the treatment or doesn't have a solid sense of trust with you.

In developing a relationship with an existing or a new patient, ask questions and listen to hear and to understand the concerns, the likes and dislikes. When you can sense the patient's needs, you can meet them where they are coming from. The most important thing you will do during your initial interview is establish the patient's motivator—his/her emotional *hot button*. Know that a person will make a purchase based on "what's in this for me", or "how will this benefit me", or "how will this purchase help me".

Remember to be flexible. Sense the patients' needs. Meet them "where they are coming from." Don't be too directive; don't be judgmental. Don't X-ray a person's pocketbook. Listen. Present the dentistry that you believe will meet the patient's needs. Make the financing of the dentistry comfortable by

**Tips
To Bank
On**

*Don't X-ray a person's
pocketbook.*

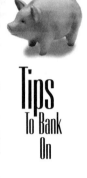

offering several options. Then, get out of the way and let the patient make his/her own decision about his/her health, well-being, and appearance.

If the patient doesn't say "when do we start", you presented the fee too soon. You do not present the fee until motivators are determined, all clinical questions are answered, and the person wants the dentistry. "A person will buy what they want long before they will buy what they need". You *must* determine the motivators and present to that motivator. Trying to "close" too early is as non-productive as not closing at all.

LISTEN YOUR WAY TO FINANCIAL ACCEPTANCE

Listen your way to financial acceptance? How? Is this possible? Don't you have to talk and talk and talk before a person will understand things well enough to say "yes"? No. Listening may be the single most important communication skill that you can access when you are trying to establish that relationship with a patient and when you are trying to gain insight into their person concerns. Listening can make a positive difference in your dental practice.

There are four different activities that a person does with his/her language—reading, writing, speaking, and listening. Most people say that listening is the most powerful of all these skills. However, most people also agree that of these four communication skills that listening is the skill that needs the most work and attention.

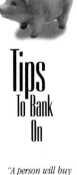

Kevin Murphy, President of CDK Management and Consulting Associates, says that listening is 1) the accurate perception of what is being communicated, 2) a process in perpetual motion, 3) a two-way exchange in which both parties involved must always be receptive to the thoughts, ideas, and emotions of the other.

Mr. Murphy also says that "Listening is a natural process that goes against human nature"!

WHAT GETS IN THE WAY OF EFFECTIVE LISTENING IN THE DENTAL OFFICE?

Some of the prevalent deterrents to good listening in your office may be:

- time pressure

- stress — not being able to relax,

- mind set — being rigid in thought processes,

- talking too much — dominating the conversation as the "authority",

- thinking what to say in response, instead of listening,

- lack of interest.

Before you can learn how to listen effectively, you must develop an understanding of the attitudes necessary for listening to take place. An open mind is necessary for the skill of listening to be considered a true avenue of communication.

By listening to your patients you will learn how they feel about your services, and you will learn what it is they want. Then you will be better able to meet those needs. The patient wins and you, the dental team, win with increased productivity.

WHAT ATTITUDES ARE REQUIRED FOR SUCCESSFUL LISTENING TO TAKE PLACE

1) **You must want to hear what the other person is saying.**

This takes time! Scheduled time for discussion of financial issues lets you and the patient focus on this intimate discussion, without interruption. The patient won't feel rushed and neither will you. You must have time if you are going to listen well enough to determine a person's questions, concerns, and particular needs. The point here is vital: You must be able to hear the other person's point of view— determine what they want, then be able to communicate well enough to answer those wants.

2) You must sincerely want to help the other person with the problem.

The position of financial coordinator must be assigned to someone who *wants* to deal with this area. This takes a confident person, one who (a) believes in the benefits of dental care, (b) has faith in the dentist's ability, (c) can quote total treatment fees without flinching, (d) is an excellent communicator—one who can "listen".

3) You must be able to accept the other person's true feelings.

Other people will have feelings different from yours; sometimes these feelings may be different from what you think they *should* be! Learning to accept these differences and not letting that difference affect your relationship to that person takes time and effort!

In the area of financing, you may hear statements from patients that could be offensive. For example: "This fee is ridiculous. What does that dentist want to do—go to Hawaii on my mouth?" and so on.

I've heard everything—you probably have also. It may be difficult to accept another person's opinion at first. As difficult as it may be to listen to the person, letting the patient get things out on the table and making sure you are clear as to where they are coming from is the first step to getting to a financial agreement.

4) You must trust that the other person has the ability to handle his/her feelings.

You cannot make another person feel differently. However, you can influence a person's opinion. That's what you want—the opportunity to influence a person's opinion. You want to get the patient to a place

Tips To Bank On

You must be able to hear the other person's point of view— determine what they want, then be able to communicate well enough to answer those wants.

where he/she will listen to you—listen to the options you have available for payment. The only way to get a person to listen to you is to listen to them first.

The goal of determining open lines of communication is to develop a win/win solution—one that is good for the patient and one that is good for the practice. In order to develop a financial solution with a patient you must establish the needs of both parties— what does the patient need? What does the practice need? A good solution is one that works for both parties.

5) **You must know that, many times, feelings are transitory.**

Be accepting of the "human nature" of changing feelings. Don't make judgments about a person based on your automatic reaction. Take the time to truly define the problem, design a plan for the resolution of the problem, implement the solution.

Don't pre-judge anyone. You may be surprised at which patients accept the full treatment plan. If you go into every financial presentation with a positive mindset and if you *think* that the person will accept the treatment, you will have a much greater acceptance rate.

6) **You must be able to actually listen without becoming self-stimulated or defensive.**

Allow for a *separateness*. The other person is unique from you and responds in his/her own way. Respect this separateness. i.e., Often, when you *hear* what another person says, you *do* become defensive and, thus, close the door to *good communication*. A more effective way to truly *listen* to another is to reflect back to the person what you think you are hearing. By *actively listening* to a person you are able to get to the center of the message—what the sender really means.

Saying nothing at all *does* communicate acceptance, if you are truly *listening attentively*. Silence is a nonverbal message that, when used effectively, can make a person feel genuinely accepted. Ask a question. Then give the patient your full attention through good body language—eye contact, being on the same level, slightly leaning forward, arms and legs uncrossed.

When a person begins to share information with you, deliver simple responses like, "Oh", "I see", "Really", Uh huh" and so on. These simple *passive listening* responses encourage a person to *go on* and to give you more information—which is what you need and want—more information. Remember, you want information so that you can determine where the person is coming from. Let the patient give you the lead. Then take the lead and engineer your presentation to follow that lead.

ACTIVE LISTENING

When a situation, or problem, warrants a more active participation by both parties, the communication skill called *active listening* is constructively applicable. Active listening is the restating in your own words what you understand the other person to be saying. In actively listening to someone, you need to give careful attention to both the content of the message and to the feeling that is being transmitted.

Example

Financial Coordinator: "Ms. Jones, the fee for the recommended treatment is $500. How would you like to take care of that?"

Patient: "You have got to be kidding! For one tooth?"

Financial Coordinator: "You seem surprised with the fee."

Patient: "I am. I can't believe that it costs that much to fix this tooth. I just think I'll have him pull it out."

Financial Coordinator: "You feel that the fee is too high? Or are you not interested in saving your tooth?"

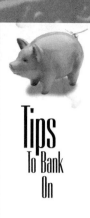

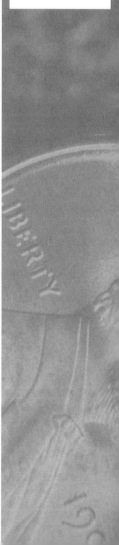

Feed back to the person your own understanding of their message. This type of listening helps to establish clarity. You must know the concern of the patient. In the above example, the financial coordinator is determining if the patient is not interested in her health or if she is concerned about that fee. If she is concerned about the fee—she then will want to find out if the problem is the total fee or if she simply needs a way to pay for the treatment.

You will shoot yourself in the foot if you begin answering questions before you determine the *real* problem. Often the opening remarks are only the peripheral issue. Listening lets you peel the layers of the situation to get to the core, the real issue.

Tips To Bank On

Listening lets you peel the layers of the situation to get to the core, the real issue.

DON'T BECOME DEFENSIVE

Although there are many roadblocks that get in the way of good listening, becoming defensive toward the other person is, perhaps, the greatest barrier. When a person becomes defensive, the lines of communication close. Therefore, when discussing possible treatment—and certainly when discussing financing—becoming defensive is detrimental.

In order *not* to become defensive, the single best skill you can use is listening. According to Dr. Thomas Gordon in his book, *Leader Effectiveness Training,* there are three characteristics that describe a good listener:

1. Empathy

2. Genuineness

3. Acceptance

Native American lore says that "You can't walk a mile in another person's moccasins unless you first take off your own". That's a good way to describe *empathy.* The only way to let a person know that you are really interested in him/her, without judgment, is to listen to them. A person feels important, respected, and validated when you listen.

Genuineness means that you are congruent or sincere in your willingness to hear what another person is thinking and feeling. It also means that you are willing to be honest with your own feelings.

Acceptance. You may not agree with what another person says, but you must be able to accept their opinion or, at least, accept their right to express their opinion.

However, if the relationship is established and strong, you *can* impact the person's opinion because he/she will listen to you. If you listen to, validate, and respect that person—you will get that right back. In order for the patient to listen to your financial presentation, he/she must respect you. In order to respect you, you must have first established respect for them through listening.

When you learn to integrate active listening into your repertoire of communication skills you truly involve the mind in a dynamic process, rather than using only the ears in a physical process. You reach out to the sender of the message with your own message of caring and acceptance. If you use only your ears to "hear" the words, but do not use your mind actively to understand *what* is really being said and felt, then you do nothing to advance communication. The result is *failure to communicate!*

From active listening feedback, the sender gets tangible evidence of how the receiver deciphered the message. The sender can either confirm the accuracy of the message ("yes, that is just what I meant.") or can deny the accuracy ("no, that's not what I meant at all. It's like this . . .") This kind of continual feedback allows us to be absolutely sure that we understand what is being said. This also provides a sense of *empathy* and *acceptance* for the one delivering the message.

LISTEN, LISTEN, LISTEN

You've heard the saying, "God gave you two ears and one mouth so that you could listen twice as much as you talk". Pretty good advice.

Tips To Bank On

"God gave you two ears and one mouth so that you could listen twice as much as you talk".

No matter what the specific goals and objectives of your practice, every one of your days is an exchange of context and emotion—that *is* communication—both verbal and non-verbal. If you choose to ignore or underplay this constant exchange of data, you will be missing an incredible opportunity to expand your practice by utilizing numerous information sources, by solving everyday problems constructively and painlessly, by drawing upon the talent that penetrates your practice every day! Put the greatest single management tool you can possess—*listening*—into effect. Put it to work *for* you!

PRESENTATION OF THE FEE

How do you move from the clinical presentation to the financial presentation? How does the dentist keep the doors open for a good financial discussion—but not get involved with that discussion?

Once the dentist has presented his/her recommendations , he/she needs to ask the following question:

> **Dr:** "Ms. Jones, do you have any questions regarding the treatment that I have just presented to you?"
>
> (She may say "no". However, if she says anything about money, like . . .)
>
> **Patient:** "Well, yes, I do have a couple of questions. How much is this, and how can I pay for it?"
>
> (Then, the dentist should answer in the following way:)
>
> **Dr.:** "Ms. Jones, are you concerned about the financing of the dentistry?"
>
> **Patient:** "Yes. It sounds like a lot of treatment, and I'm not sure I can afford it."
>
> **Dr.:** "I certainly understand how you feel. Many patients have felt the same concern until they found out

that we do have several excellent payment options. Jan, our financial coordinator, will discuss the total investment and will tell you about those options. She is very competent, and I feel confident that she will be able to work things out for you. If the two of you are able to develop a financial arrangement that works for you is this the type of dental treatment you would like to receive?

Patient: "Yes. I know I need this. And I want to do it. I just need to see what it's going to cost."

Dr.: "OK. Then, I will excuse myself and let you and Jan work together. I am certain that you will find a comfortable option, and I will look forward to working with you to get you healthy again."

The above discussion is a closing sequence by the dentist that clarifies whether or not there are clinical questions that he/she needs to address. It also leads nicely into the financial discussion. It paves the way for the financial coordinator to take over and to do so with the professional compliment of the dentist, thus building the patient's confidence in her and in her ability. The dentist acknowledges the patient's concern but does not get involved in the financial presentation.

I do not have a problem with the dentist quoting the fee. However, the financial coordinator needs to be the one who makes the financial arrangement.

Notice that the dentist *did* open the door for the discussion by telling the patient that there were several financial options available, but the dentist *did not* discuss those options. The dentist needs to get back to the chair. Also, the business person will do a better job and she will be less vulnerable tthan the dentist to requests by the patient to let them pay out their dentistry at $2.00 per month for the rest of their lives.

Now the financial/treatment coordinator changes her location. She can sit where the dentist was sitting before his/her departure. She needs to be sitting on the same level with the patient and there should not be anything between them like a big desk. Sitting next to each other or sitting at either side of a corner of a table is ideal. Body language is critical. Again, you want everything to be advantageous for the very best presentation/discussion to take place.

Financial Coordinator: "Ms. Jones, I know that Dr. Jameson asked if you had any questions about the treatment that he recommended and you said no, but I thought that there might be something you would like to ask me about the treatment before we discuss the financial responsibility."

Patient: "No. He explained everything real well. And I could see the problems on that camera. So, hit me with the tough stuff."

FC: "The fee for the treatment that Dr. Jameson has recommended is $3000. How would you like to take care of that?"

(This is exactly how you present the fee: the statement of the total investment followed by the *qualifying question,* "How would you like to take care of that?" Let your patient give you the lead. You stay in control of a conversation by asking questions. Ask this question. Then, be quiet and listen to the patient's response. They will give you the direction you need to find the right solution.)

Patient: "Three thousand dollars! You have got to be kidding? "

FC: "It seems that you are surprised with that figure."

(Actively listen to the patient to see if you are hearing them accurately. Active listening is reflecting back to the person your perception of the message they have just sent. This gives you a chance to clarify. Do not overreact. Do not start back pedaling. Just listen.)

Patient: "Surprised isn't the word for it. I'm shocked! I had no idea it would be that much. That's way too much money for teeth!"

FC: "How much too much is this for you?"

(The answer to the statement "That costs too much" needs a responsive question. The FC wants to know if the whole thing is too much—or if the treatment is just more than had been expected. Again, with a qualifying question, she gains necessary information to move ahead.)

Patient: "Oh, about twice too much! I knew it would be quite a bit, but $3000!"

(Here the question asked by the FC led to the patient's response that the total investment wasn't the shock, it was the amount over what she was prepared to pay. In addition to clarifying how much too much she felt the investment would be, the FC made note of the fact that the patient had come in knowing that there would be quite a bit of treatment and that there would be an investment. But she thinks it is about twice too much—about $1500 too much.)

FC: "Ms. Jones, if I am hearing you correctly, you are saying that you were prepared to pay approximately $1500 for your treatment and that the other $1500 is the real stumbling block. Am I right about that?"

(Clarification through active listening)

Patient: "Yeah. I guess so. I had some money saved for this, but not that much."

FC: "Ms. Jones, since you are prepared to pay $1500 of the treatment from your savings account, if we are able to finance the other $1500 so that the investment is not a financial burden for you, would that make it possible for us to go ahead?"

(Here the FC is trying to get back to an open line of communication with the patient. She is trying to get past the issue of the total investment and have the patient start thinking of a method of payment that would let her proceed with treatment. If the patient's mind is closed, she can hear no further discussion. The mind must be reopened so that a logical discussion can take place. If a person is overwhelmed with emotion, they cannot think logically.)

Patient: "Well, maybe. What can you do?"

FC: "If there were any way that you could pay for the treatment in advance, we would reduce your fee by 5%. We would not be involved with any bookkeeping and that would save us time and money and we would be able to pass those savings on to you. In your situation, that would save you $150. That's quite a bit of savings. Does that sound like a possibility?"

(You will notice that she closes her statements with a question to get the patient's response and to keep the patient involved.)

Patient: "No. I have the $1500 cash, but no more than that."

FC: "We could spread the $1500 difference equally throughout your treatment. The doctor will be seeing you for three separate visits. We could accept three $500 payments with one payment being due at each of your three appointments."

Patient: "No. That is still too much for me. I have a limited income and can't do $500 at a time. Can I just make payments to you for a while?"

FC: "What you would like to do is take care of the $1500 right now and then spread out the remainder of the fee over a period of time and keep the payments small, is that right?"

(Active Listening)

Patient: "Yeah. That's the only way I could do it."

FC: "How much per month would you be willing and able to invest?"

(This is a critical question. The FC is, again, qualifying. She needs to ask this question to see which type of payment option she will offer in order to satisfy the patient's need.)

Patient: "Oh, I was thinking about maybe $40 or $50 per month."

FC: "I am happy to tell you that we do have a couple of options that will let you do just that. We accept VISA,

111

Mastercard, or Discover. We could place the $1500 balance on one of those bank cards—whichever one you choose—and then you could pay however much you want every month. Does that work for you?"

Patient: "No. I already have those maxed out. I don't want to use a credit card."

FC: "Then, Ms. Jones, let me tell you about another option that many of our patients have chosen to use. We have an arrangement with a financing company called, ABC Financing Company. They offer a financing program for healthcare. You apply right here in our office. You don't have to go anywhere. The application is easy to complete and I will be more than happy to assist you.

We will fax the application to ABC and once they have extended a line of credit to you, we can go ahead with your dental care, finance the $1500 and your monthly payments will be around $35—$40 per month. So, what I am saying is that for less than $50 per month, you can receive the care that Dr. Jameson has recommended and you will be able to comfortably fit the monthly payments into your family situation. How does that sound?"

Patient: "OK. That sounds pretty good. "

FC: "Great. I have an application right here. Let's work together to fill this out."

Study the verbal skills that I outlined in chapter three and here on how to present a healthcare financing program—and how to overcome the normal objections that will come up. Practice. Practice. Practice. You should be able to answer any objection. The verbal skills should roll off your tongue because you have learned them so well.

Do not let yourself be placed in a position to become flustered because you don't know how to respond to a patient's objection. If you believe in your services, in the payment options you have available, and if you have the verbal skills mastered, your confidence will be assured.

Once the financial agreement has been made, write it down. The patient may keep a copy for their own reference and records. You file one in the patient's chart. Know that just because someone tells you they understand—or that they will remember—doesn't mean that they will. Your records will become vital.

Every time a person comes to the office, you will be collecting the agreed upon amount of money. You will, also, know the method of payment selected and be prepared for the collection process. Once the fee for the day has been collected, remind or reconfirm the patient's financial responsibility for the next visit.

No one should ever walk out of your door without an appointment either with the hygienist for continuous care or with the dentist for the next phase of restorative care—or in some cases—both. In addition, no one should ever walk out your door without being very clear about their financial responsibility for the next visit.

Tips To Bank On

Know that just because someone tells you they understand—or that they will remember—doesn't mean that they will. Your records will become vital.

SAMPLE SCRIPTS FOR HANDLING FINANCIAL QUESTIONS

You need to be ready for patient's questions regarding your financial program. Here are some suggested scripts for such questions, as well as some suggested responses to challenging financial situations.

Example: You are no longer handling long term accounts on your own books.

"Ms. Jones, we are no longer able to carry accounts on our own books over a long period of time. Our accountant no longer will allow us to manage a banking business within our practice. We have found that in order to maintain comfortable fees for our patients that we must be able to concentrate our time and money on our dental care."

Example: Patient wants to wait until after insurance has paid to make any private payments.

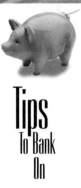

Tips To Bank On

. . . no one should ever walk out your door without being very clear about their financial responsibility for the next visit.

"Ms. Jones, I can understand that you want to see what your insurance will pay before you make any investment yourself. However, because we have accurate information on your insurance benefits, we are able to estimate very closely what your insurance probably will cover and the portion for which you will be responsible. Therefore, in order to cover our laboratory and operating expenses, we ask that you take care of your part at the time of the service.

We will file your insurance as a service to you. However, if for any reason your insurance company does not pay what we expect, then you will be responsible for the balance."

Example: Patient says that they don't get paid until next week. Can they send you a check?

"Ms. Jones, I can accept a postdated check. I will keep it here and will not deposit the check until next Friday."

Example: Patient doesn't have her checkbook!

"Oh, I see. Well, that happens sometimes, doesn't it? We do accept MasterCard, Visa and Discover. Which would you prefer? You don't have these cards? Well, then I will give you a statement and a self addressed, stamped envelope. You can send us a check as soon as you get home. We will look forward to receiving that check in a couple of days." (Make a note in the tickler file. If you don't get the check in a few days, call.)

Example: You have made financial arrangements with a person. They come in the day of the preparation appointment. When they are being excused from the clinical area, they inform you that they do not have the agreed upon payment.

"Ms. Jones, I am confused. We discussed your financial responsibility for this appointment and came to a comfortable agreement. However, since we do not carry accounts on our own books, I would be able to accept a credit card payment today. Then, we will be able to send the models of your case to the laboratory."

If they don't have a bank card, tell them you will hold the case and as soon as they bring in payment, you will send it to the lab.

VERBAL SKILLS TO
USE WHEN DISCUSSING FINANCING

As I have said throughout this book, the way you say something makes all the difference in the world and your success will be in direct proportion to your ability to communicate. There are some words that bring about a positive response and some that seem to stimulate a negative response. Several of these are listed. Get used to using the positive words and phrases and eliminate the others.

Words and Phrases:

Negative	Positive
Money, Dollars,	Fee For the Service
Charge, Cost	Financial Responsibility Total Investment Monthly Investment
Bill	Statement
Discount	Cash Courtesy/Fee Reduction/Accounting Reduction
Sign here	Please initial May I ask for your signature
Policy	Financial options
Deposit	Initial investment
Do you want to pay today?	Mrs. Jones, your fee today is Fifty-five Will that be cash, check, or do you prefer to use a bank card?

Exercise

Develop scripts of verbal skills that would be appropriate and effective for handling the following situations:

1. A financial arrangement is made for treatment. The patient is in the middle of the treatment but is not abiding by the financial agreement.

   _____

   _____

2. You have made a financial arrangement that is comfortable for your patient and for you. However, the patient has not fulfilled his obligations. You have made consistent efforts to negotiate an agreement but have not received cooperation from the patient. Now you are making your last telephone call before you turn the patient over for legal action. You wish to make one last effort to prevent such action.

   _____

   _____

   _____

Possible Responses

1. "Ms. Jones, I became concerned when we didn't receive your payments as scheduled, because this may force us to delay your treatment. I know you want to proceed with your treatment and complete it this year. And so, it is critical that we come to an agreement so that you can go ahead with your dentistry."

2. "Ms. Jones, I will be forced to turn your account over for legal action unless I receive your payment in full immediately. I am calling today to discuss this with you in the hopes that we might be able to do something about the account so that we can avoid this legal action. I'm sure you would agree with me that avoiding such action would be better for both of us."

SUMMARY

The making of the financial arrangement is one of the most important moments in your time with a patient. Without question a person's willingness to *go ahead* may depend on your ability to define their situation and/or problems and to work out a solution.

As good as you present the financial responsibility and the options available for payment, there will still be objections. Objections are not to be avoided or to be feared. An objection can be a door opener for you and may prove to be extremely valuable.

Let's look at how to handle the normal objection of cost.

Overcoming the Fear of Cost: Handling Objections

*"It costs 5–6 times more to win
a new customer than it does to keep one."*

— MICHAEL LE BOEUF, PH.D.
FAST FORWARD

"**W**ell, Doctor, I'd like to go ahead with this treatment. I know I need it. But it just costs too much! I can't afford it right now. I'll just have to wait."

Have you heard this before? Does the response ever come at the completion of your excellent presentation of recommendations?

Do you get discouraged? Do you wonder what you can do to deal with the objection, the barrier, the fear of cost?

Let's look at a step by step way to handle objections, specifically the objection of *cost*.

Tips To Bank On

Your entire team must believe in the services you are providing.

1. VALIDATE YOUR SERVICES AND YOUR QUALITY TO YOURSELVES.

Do you feel that the value of your services exceeds the fee you are asking for it? Before *anything* else happens, you must convince yourself of your own worth.

Key Point

- Your entire team must believe in the services you are providing.

- You must have a strong commitment to your work and to the patients you serve.

- You, as care providers, add value to the lives of those people.

- Make sure that the treatment your patients are receiving is an equitable exchange for the fee. Thus: value = value

Exercise

List the services you provide for your patients—from the initial contact through the entire treatment. Now as a team, answer the following questions:

    a. What makes your services *special?*

    b. What *added value* touches do you provide that make your practice unique?

    c. What do you do that goes beyond the expected?

2. VALIDATE YOURSELF PERSONALLY TO YOUR PATIENTS.

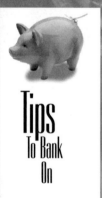

Tips To Bank On

You must establish a relationship of trust and confidence with a patient before treatment acceptance will result.

Key Point

You must establish a relationship of trust and confidence with a patient before treatment acceptance will result. Your *on going* internal marketing program should have this as its foundation. In planning your marketing/educational program, ask this question, "Does this marketing tool make a statement (consciously or subconsciously) about who we are, what we do, what our purpose is about? If the answer is *yes,* then the marketing tool is probably going to serve your purpose well. If the answer is *no,* then you may need to rethink the project.

3. VALIDATE YOUR SERVICES.

In your efforts to validate your services to existing and potential clients, do the following:

1. Use testimonial letters from enthusiastic patients.

2. Use before and after photographs of *your* patients to illustrate a particular service you provide. (Be sure to obtain written permission from your patient).

3. Provide civic presentations throughout your community using before and after slides of treatment you have provided.

    a. Concentrate on one subject at a time i.e., cosmetic dentistry, non-surgical periodontal therapy, preventive dentistry, etc.

    b. The program must not be self serving—but, rather, educational.

    c. Leave a written piece with each participant.

    d. Keep the program short, 20–30 minutes.

    e. Use layman's language.

    f. Use visual aids—slides are excellent.

    g. Be enthusiastic and energetic.

4. Make sure that every aspect of your practice epitomizes the professional image you wish to project.

All of these foundational efforts work to establish a value for the service that far outweighs the *fee.*

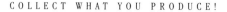

Key Point

You want to have the exchange of value be equitable—but perceived to tilt in the favor of the patient.

HANDLING OBJECTIONS

Tom Hopkins of Scottsdale, Arizona is one of the nation's leading sales trainers. I have had the privilege of studying with Mr. Hopkins and he has totally changed my attitude about objections. I used to dread an objection. Why? Because I *assumed* that if a person objected—in this case to the cost of the dentistry or to our financial options—that they didn't want to have the dentistry at all. I felt terrible because I thought an objection meant that the person was upset or irritated. Avoidance of a controversial issue seemed to be a good way to get out of feeling uncomfortable.

Then, I studied with Tom Hopkins and learned that an objection—including the objection of cost—is actually a step forward in completing an agreement. If your patients do *not* pose any objections or raise any questions, they're probably not interested. In other words, I learned to look forward to an objection because that meant that the person was interested. That's what we want. Now I know that an objection is a gift.

Four Insights About Objections:

1. You identify an objection by asking questions and listening.

2. An objection is a request for further information.

3. If a person presents an objection that means that he/she is interested.

4. Objections are the steps necessary to the close.

An objection is actually an opportunity for you. It defines a specific area of concern. You will need to ask questions to isolate or identify what objections, if any, might get in the way of a person going ahead with treatment.

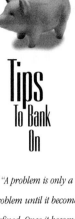

Key Point

"A problem is only a problem until it becomes defined. Once it becomes defined it becomes manageable".

When an objection is posed by a patient, take the following steps:

- **Hear Out The Objection.** Don't interrupt. Encourage the person to express himself. Objections often diminish when a person is allowed to talk about it. In addition, this gives you another chance to listen, to show concern, to empathize (not sympathize), and to let the person sense your understanding. Thus, you *validate* your patient!

- **Actively Listen.** Rephrase and repeat back to the person what you think you have heard them say. This gives you a chance to 1) clarify 2) reinforce the patient and 3) move forward.

- **Reinforce the Importance of the Objection.** *There's no benefit to disagreeing with or arguing with a patient.* When you listen to the concerns, reinforce those concerns, share in the development of possible solutions, you will be less likely to see that patient leave without scheduling an appointment.

Example

> **Patient:** "I don't want to lose my teeth, but I sure don't want to spend this much money if this isn't going to last."
>
> **Dentist:** "Keeping your teeth for a lifetime is important to you, and you want to make sure that the investment you make is going to be one that lasts for as long as possible."
>
> **Patient:** "Yes".
>
> **Dentist:** "I totally agree with you."

- **Answer the Objection.** Provide further education. Stress the end results and benefits of the treatment you

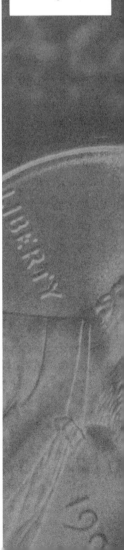

Tips To Bank On

"A problem is only a problem until it becomes defined. Once it becomes defined it becomes manageable".

are recommending. Turn the objection into a benefit. Establish value. Use the "feel, felt, found" response:

> "Mr. Patient, I understand how you feel. Many patients have felt the same concern about making an investment in comprehensive dental care, until they found out that an investment in quality, comprehensive care *now* will 1) provide better health 2) last longer 3) look better and 4) save money in the long run."

- **Confirm the Answer.** Get the patient involved with you by asking questions. Then stop and wait for the response. This involvement helps a patient to feel an active part of the decision making process. And that's *exactly* what you want!

> **Dentist:** "This type of comprehensive care provided now would answer your concern about making a stable, long term investment, wouldn't it?"

- **Change the Direction of the Conversation—Move Forward.** Using a phrase, such as *by the way,* change the flow of focus of the conversation. Move to another area of interest that will move the conversation in a positive direction. Such as,

> **Dentist:** "By the way, Mr. Patient, do you have any particular scheduling concerns that we need to be aware of?"

- **Close.** Once you have dealt with the objections, ask for a commitment—*close.* Closing an agreement means *asking!* If you don't ask for a commitment, you are giving your patient permission to procrastinate!

> **Dentist:** "Mr. Patient, do you have any further questions about the treatment that I am

Tips
To Bank
On

If you don't ask for a commitment, you are giving your patient permission to procrastinate!

recommending for you—any questions about the clinical aspects of the treatment?"

Mr. Patient: "No. I can see what is wrong and what you need to do."

Dentist: "Then, if you and Jan are able to develop a financial agreement that works for you, shall we go ahead and schedule an appointment to begin?"

Mr. Patient: "I guess so. Might as well go for it."

There is the dentist's close. Now the financial coordinator will need to do the same thing. She will reconfirm the dentistry, present the total fee, the options for payment, get a commitment for one of those options (or a combination of options), and will close. Then, she will schedule that first appointment.

Remember that you control a conversation with questions. When a person poses an objection—don't freeze up and feel that you've hit a dead end. Not so! As you skillfully learn to handle objections you will find that these objections are progressive steps taken to *move ahead.*

Key Point

If you *know* something is going to be brought up as an objection, *you* bring it up. This gives you an opportunity to turn a potential negative into a positive.

Example

Dentist: "Mr. Patient, before I give you the results of my analysis, and before I explain the treatment I recommend for you to reach optimum oral health, first let me tell you that if you have any concerns about the financing of your treatment, we do have convenient, long-term financing right here in our office. I tell you this so that, for now, we can both concentrate on your treatment. But please know that we will discuss financial options in full. We want to make sure that you are clear and comfortable with this important part of your treatment. OK?"

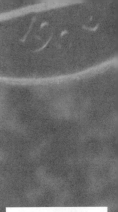

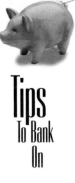

Tips
To Bank On

If you know *something is going to be brought up as an objection, you bring it up. This gives you an opportunity to turn a potential negative into a positive.*

EXAMPLES OF CLOSING SEQUENCES

Dentist: "And so, Mr. Patient, the financing of the dentistry is a concern for you, is that right?"

Patient: "Yes"

Dentist: "If we are able to find a financial solution you would like to proceed, right?"

or

Dentist: "Mr. Patient, if I understand you correctly, this is the type of dentistry you would like to receive."

Patient: "Yes, it is."

Dentist: "Then, if we are able to make the financing of the dentistry comfortable for you, is there any reason why we shouldn't go ahead and schedule an appointment to begin your treatment?"

or

Dentist: "Now that we have agreed on the treatment that you will receive and once Jan has worked out the details of your financial agreement, we will schedule you first appointment and go ahead. How does that sound?"

LEARNING TO HANDLE OBJECTIONS

Objections diminish when a person is allowed and encouraged to talk about them. And so,

1. Restate the patient's wants and needs.

2. Actively listen to their concerns. Rephrase and feed back their objections.

3. Validate the person by using the "Feel, Felt, Found".

4. Turn the patient's objections around by asking a question to establish value.

5. Encourage the patient to share with you in the development of a solution.

Key Point

"If a person is allowed to be a part of a decision-making process, he/she will be more likely to buy into the decision."

You can't push anyone into making a decision, but you can lead them carefully and caringly by asking questions and listening. You can't *talk* people into going ahead but you can *listen* them into *going ahead*.

ONE MORE TIME:
EXAMPLES OF VERBAL SKILLS THAT
IDENTIFY AND OVERCOME OBJECTIONS

A person says, "That's just too much."

When a person tells you the fee is too much, actively listen to make sure you're hearing them correctly.

> **Dentist/Business Manager:** "You feel the fee is too high for the services I'm recommending for you? Or is the investment difficult for you at this time?"

> **Patient:** "I'm sure the treatment is worth the fee, but I can't afford this right now."

> **Dentist/Business Manager:** "Tell me, Mr. Patient, if we can make the financing comfortable for you with a convenient monthly payment plan, would this make it possible for you to proceed?"

> **Patient:** "Probably."

> **Dentist/Business Manager:** "How much per month could you invest?"

His answer to this question would let you know if you could *go ahead* by offering him MasterCard, VISA, Discover, or a HealthCare Financing Program.

Tips To Bank On

You can't push anyone into making a decision, but you can lead them carefully and caringly by asking questions and listening.

Example

> **Patient:** "Gee, Doctor, I want those veneers. I hate my smile. But $3000 is just too much!

> **Dentist/Business Manager:** "How much too much is that, Mr. Patient?"

> **Patient:** "About $1500 too much. I saved $1500 for this—but, wow, I had no idea it would be this much!"

> **Dentist/Business Manager:** "So, the solution we're looking for is a way to finance the $1500 beyond your current savings, is that right?"

> **Patient:** "Yes."

Now you know that the $3000 isn't the problem, it's the $1500 that needs attention and assistance.

Example

> **Patient:** "I'll have to think this over."

> **Dentist or Financial Coordinator:** "Well, I appreciate that, Ms. Patient. I know you wouldn't take the time to think this over if you weren't interested. So that I can make sure that I am clear, won't you please tell me, what is it that you need to think about? Is it whether or not this is the type of treatment that would be best for you?"

> **Patient:** "Oh, no. I know that I need this."

> **Dentist or Financial Coordinator:** "Then do you need to think about whether or not I/Dr. Jameson would be the one to provide that treatment?"

> **Patient:** "No, if I do this, I want you to do it. I don't want anyone else to stick their hands in my mouth!"

> **Dentist or Financial Coordinator:** "Then, tell me Ms. Patient, is it the money? Do you need to think about whether or not you are able to make this investment now?"

Patient: "Yeah. Money is a bit tight right now."

What has happened in this example is that because of careful and caring questioning, the true problem has been identified and can now be addressed. The communication skills here make it comfortable and possible for the patient to say that they need to find a way to pay for the treatment. Many times a patient will say that they need to "think it over" and the dental person with whom they are conversing will just say, "Oh, OK. Well, give us a call when you are ready."

At that moment, the whole issue drops in a bucket. You must identify what the problem is for the patient. You must make it comfortable for him/her to tell you if there is a financial issue. Some people are embarrassed or too proud to come out and tell you that they need some financial help. Let the patient know that you understand the situation, and that you have alternatives. Open doors that historically have been closed.

Example

Patient: "I can't believe I need this much work! How is this possible?"

Dentist or Financial Coordinator: "I can't tell you that, Mr. Patient. There are many things that affect your oral health: age, nutrition—what and how you eat, home care, stress. Have you been under stress over the last year or so?"

Patient: "Man, have I!"

Dentist or Financial Coordinator: "Our responsibility is to evaluate your situation and make a thorough diagnosis based on a comprehensive gathering of data and a complete analysis of that data. Then, after careful study, make recommendations that we believe would help you to get and maintain oral health for a lifetime. And that's what we have done. You have total control in the decision making. Whether or not you proceed with the treatment that I/we are recommending is completely up to you and the choice is yours alone. However, my/our responsibility as your

129

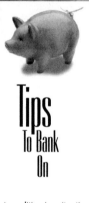

Tips
To Bank
On

An objection is a request for further information and shows that the person is interested in a continued discussion of the proposal.

Tips
To Bank
On

A condition is a situation that is going on in a person's life that absolutely prevents them from going ahead—at least for the moment.

dentist/dental team is to do the very best job we can to diagnose, treatment plan, and present to you a course of action that we believe would be in your best interest. Is that OK with you?"

Tom Hopkins has taught me the difference between an objection and a condition. My understanding of this difference has been very helpful as I work with people—whether in the dental office or elsewhere.

An objection is a request for further information and shows that the person is interested in a continued discussion of the proposal.

A condition is a situation that is going on in a person's life that absolutely prevents them from going ahead—at least for the moment. Say that a person has just been released from the hospital and has high bills there or that a person has lost a job or has four kids in college. All of these are conditions that might prevent him/her from accepting treatment. However, it doesn't mean that he/she doesn't want it!

You are responsibile for doing the very best job you can of diagnosing, treatment planning, and presenting the dentistry. Make the financing of the dentistry as comfortable as you can and then get out of the way and let the patient make his/her own decision.

As you are presenting, ask closing questions that will identify objections—or in some cases—conditions. If you identify a condition, let the patient know that you will be there when he/she is ready and that you will stay in touch. Knowing the difference between a condition and an objection lets you know where to go and how to get there. The communciation skills for this type of identification are critical. The very best way to identify a condition or an objection is by asking questions and listening—actively!

Here is an Exercise for you. Practice will give you the necessary confidence to communicate financially.

1. List the main financial barriers or objections your patients give to you.

2. Using the skills from this chapter, formulate scripts that will help you deal with and overcome those objections.

3. Role play using these scripts.

4. After the role playing, answer these questions.

    a. Did I listen carefully?

    b. Did I repeat what I thought were the patient's main concerns?

    c. Did I validate the patient?

    d. Did I answer each objection with a *values* question?

    e. Did I go through the steps of dealing with an objection?

    f. When I overcame the objections, did I close?

SUMMARY

Do not fear an objection, even the objection of money. Rather, look at this as an opportunity.

Know that, if you do your best and the person does not go ahead, they are rejecting the treatment proposal. They are *not* rejecting you.

Combine a strong belief in your team and the services you provide with the skills to get that message across. Then you can deal effectively with, "Gee, Doc, it costs too much!"

Financing Cosmetic Dentistry

7

*"Once you decide to have
cosmetic dentistry, you can work out
the best method of paying for it."*

— DR. RON GOLDSTEIN
CHANGE YOUR SMILE

One of the most fulfilling aspects of being a dental professional is being able to make a positive change in a person's smile—a change that will enhance a person's feeling of self worth and self confidence. The rewards of providing cosmetic dental care are many.

1. The challenge of performing highly intricate dental procedures.

2. Enhancing a person's self image.

3. Using one's artistic and clinical skills.

4. Having patients *want* to be in the chair.

5. Expressions of gratitude from patients instead of complaints.

6. Healthy revenue for the practice.

However, with few exceptions, cosmetic dental treatment will require a greater investment than $500—(there's that number again!)—the place where people begin to *balk* at the cost of treatment. So, what are your choices?

- Don't do cosmetic dentistry.

- Only do one tooth at a time.

- Carry accounts on your own books, letting patients make small monthly payments directly to you.

- Do the dentistry for free.

- Do cosmetic dentistry only on the wealthy population.

- Design payment options that will make the financing of your dental care comfortable for the majority of your patients while keeping you out of the banking business.

Of course, the last is the answer of choice. Offering the payment options recommended in chapter one will give the majority of your patients an opportunity to receive cosmetic treatment while keeping you out of the banking business. You need to be doing what you do best, providing exquisite dental artistry.

OUR OWN EXPERIENCE

John uses the services of a very large lab in the central part of the country. The manager of that lab tells me that John sends in more prescriptions for cosmetic cases than any of their other clients. They are amazed considering where John practices. In our small town of 2000 people in rural Oklahoma where our patient population is predominantly low to middle income, hard-working, salt of the earth folks, the lab cannot believe how much cosmetic dental treatment we provide.

Why is this possible in our practice? The number one reason is because John *decided* he wanted to provide this type of care. He wanted to add this to his treatment mix. In addition to quality restorative dental treatment, which he loves, he also enjoys and sees benefits of cosmetic dental treatment.

Once he *decided* to *make this happen,* we created a marketing plan to open our own doors. We are very clear about one fact: no one is going to make anything happen for us. If we want to accomplish a goal, then we must assume the responsibility to make things happen. Our decision to expand the cosmetic aspect of our practice was step one. Developing a plan of action was step two. Step three was to put the plan into action. And we are constantly evolving because of Step four— evaluating what is and is not working. If something is working, we do more of it with a commitment to continuous improvement. If something isn't working as well as we would like, then we change or alter that aspect of the plan.

The last thing we do is give up. If you want something badly enough, you will pick yourself up when you stumble or fall and you will dust yourself off to see what is still there and what has been scraped away. What is left after the healing may be a bit tougher, but it is usually stronger and better.

Wisdom comes from the tough times, not from the smooth times.

Tips To Bank On

Wisdom comes from the tough times, not from the smooth times.

EDUCATING THE POPULATION

We know that the majority of people are not aware of the fabulous opportunities that are available in dentistry today. Thus, we developed an educational program for our community and for our patient base that would introduce people to the new developments and the new possibilities.

The following strategies are a few of the segments of our marketing program. None of these strategies are new or unique, they are just good! The key to the success of any marketing program is in *just doing it*. If you are seriously interested in developing the cosmetic aspect of your practice, stop waiting for people to come in and ask you about changing their smile. Open your own doors. Pave your own way. Get serious about educating people about what's going on in dentistry and what *you* are doing to make more opportunities available.

MARKETING STRATEGIES THAT WORK

1. **Practice brochure.** In our practice brochure, there is a section in the middle of the brochure that addresses our understanding of the value of a beautiful smile. We note that we appreciate how the smile affects a person's self image. We invite people who are interested in exploring the possibility of a smile makeover to ask about cosmetic dentistry.

   These brochures are sent to all of our new patients. They are handed out at health fairs and bridal fairs where we participate two or three times per year. At these *fairs* we take one of our intra-oral cameras and show people the results of cosmetic dental treatment with before and after stored images of completed cases. In addition, at the fairs, we show a brief patient education video. We have a small VCR player that allows us to play the video continuously.

   We also give patients of record copies of our brochure to give to friends and family members who need a dental home—or who might be interested in cosmetic dentistry. We let our own patient family be our *sales force.*

2. **Patient Education Video.** In addition to showing the educational video at the health and bridal fairs, we show this video to new and existing patients who express an interest in cosmetic dentistry. There is no better way to answer questions or to stimulate interest than to show a person a video that demonstrates various situations and the solutions that are available.

3. **Patient Education Newsletters.** You have already read about my belief in patient education newsletters,

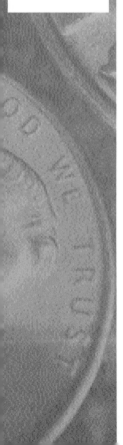

Tips
To Bank
On

Get serious about educating people about what's going on in dentistry and what you are doing to make more opportunities available.

and you have read about how we produce our own newsletter. We send this out once a quarter. We try to highlight one type of cosmetic situation or procedure in each edition or, certainly, in every other edition. Nothing that we write about in our newsletter stimulates more interest or initiates more telephone inquiries than our issues about cosmetic dentistry.

4. **Networking with Appearance Specialists.** These professionals—plastic surgeons, beauty salons, fitness centers, modeling agencies, clothing boutiques, and etc. are more than happy to network with you. You can send people their way. Or, you can provide gifts to patients who receive cosmetic treatment—gifts to receive care from one of your networking friends. They, in turn, may be willing to place your brochures or cards in their facility and may be willing to reciprocate by referring.

Tips To Bank On

See Note:

Note: Two of my clients, Dr. Joseph Miranda and Dr. Jim McLaughlin, have recently moved their practice to a wonderful location in a thriving area of Dallas, Texas. Their facility was designed with the intention of attracting patients who are interested in cosmetic dentistry. They are on the ground floor of a complex that houses numerous professional businesses. On the ground level, next door or near their own practice, is an exquisite beauty salon, a fitness center, and numerous popular restaurants.

We developed a comprehensive program to market their arrival into the building and area. A part of that program was the nurturing of a network referral system with their neighbors. The results have been exceptional. Those people who are in the appearance business understand and are interested in helping people become totally healthy and in helping them be as attractive as desired. They know that a beautiful smile is a part of the total picture.

You can do the same thing. Seek out other appearance specialists. Schedule a meeting with them. Show them before and after photographs of your cosmetic dentistry. Invite them into your office for a complimentary intra-oral camera or computer imaging session. Let these people know what you are doing in your practice to enhance a person's health and appearance. They will be amazed at the high tech equipment and at the high level of care. They will become ambassadors for you and for your practice.

5. **Brochures and Books.** Have written information—which includes photography—available in your reception area, the treatment rooms, and in the consultation area. You will want to provide written backup support for the type of treatment you are recommending in the form of educational brochures. Let patients take this material home so that they can share the information with their spouse, a friend, or family members. This may prove to be beneficial when it comes to making a decision about going ahead.

6. **Before and After Photography.** Be sure to include photography in every appointment. You will want to build your own set of before and after photographs to show people not only the features and benefits of recommended treatment but also the fact that you can produce the desired results.

7. **Intra-Oral Cameras and Imaging Systems.** There is nothing better than an intra-oral camera to show a person 'close up and personal' how their teeth and smile *really* look. A close up evaluation of the smile will give the patients a chance to tell you what they like most, what they like least, and what they would change if they could about their smile.

   With stored before and after photographs, you will be able to show patients—on the camera—examples of similar situations. They will be able to identify with these situations and see the results you were able to accomplish.

   Imaging systems, of course, let you give the patient an idea of what they can do with their own smile as you use the imager to explore possibilities.

8. **Community Presentations.** About once a month a member of our team goes to one of the civic groups in

our area and makes a 20–30 minute presentation with visual aids. We use slides to illustrate what is happening in the world of dentistry, particularly in the area of cosmetic dentistry. We have brochures about our practice and brochures about cosmetic dentistry available for handout. There is always much surprise on the part of the attendees as to what can be accomplished with new dental technology. We almost always receive a new patient who is interested in adding this dimension to his/her own life.

9. **Newspaper Articles.** We find that most newspaper editors are very interested in positive, informative articles regarding modern dentistry. We provide these articles plus photographs to the editors and tackle the subject of cosmetic dentistry as often as possible.

Also, any time a member of our team receives an award or does something special in the community, we try to get this in the newspapers. This has proven to be a tremendous source of new patients.

When our team is participating in Children's Dental Health Month, or when they are presenting a program in the community, or when John is recognized for something within the profession, we access a news release. The people in the community are proud to know that their dental professionals are active in their industry and in their community.

10. **Television and Radio.** Professionally produced spots about the practice which address cosmetic dentistry can be extremely effective. These must be produced professionally or they come across as *cheap* and are offensive rather than stimulating.

Now Just Do It

These are but a few of the many ideas that can be effective to stimulate interest in the cosmetic aspect of your practice.

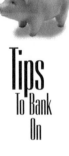

Once again, however, I must stress the fact that *nothing* is better than referrals from happy patients who recommend you because they are so pleased with the results of their own smile makeover.

In each one of our marketing strategies, we include a pleasant message about the fact that we do have comfortable financing available. We do not want to stimulate the interest in cosmetic dentistry only to have it squelched because of the fear of cost.

Overcome this potential negative before the fact. Address the issue of cost. Let people know that there are options available for payment that will make it possible for them to receive a change of smile without having to worry about how they will pay for it.

HANDLING THE OBJECTION OF COST AS IT RELATES TO COSMETIC DENTISTRY

When you are presenting your treatment recommendations, you will close your presentation by finding out if there are further questions. If not, you will ask if the patient is ready to go ahead and schedule that first appointment. (See *Great Communication = Great Production,* chapter 10, "Making an Effective Case Presentation")

Remember from our previous discussion about objections that you are serving a couple of purposes by closing: you are asking for a commitment, and you are trying to identify any objections or any barriers to treatment acceptance.

You must identify these objections before you can do anything to eliminate them. Identifying a problem is the first step in the solving of that problem.

When you have completed your presentation and are asking for the commitment, the objection of cost may emerge. That's OK. You want and need to know if this is the type of treatment a person wants, and if so what it will take to make it possible to go ahead. If the patient says that they do want this change of smile but need a way to *pay it out,* you now have a way of offering this type of financing without doing it yourself.

EXAMPLE OF FINANCIAL PRESENTATION

Financial Coordinator: "Ms. Jones, the fee for the veneers that Dr. Jameson has recommended is $4000. How would you like to take care of that?"

Ms. Jones: "Oh, I have insurance that will take care of most of it, so I'll let you find out how much they will pay, then I'll pay the difference."

Financial Coordinator: "Ms. Jones, since the treatment you will be receiving is cosmetic in nature, the insurance companies do not cover this. They consider the treatment discretionary and do not make co-payment available."

Ms. Jones: "What? I can't believe I pay this much for my insurance and it doesn't help me when I need it!"

Financial Coordinator: "I can appreciate your disappointment. However, since insurance is not a factor here, let's talk about other avenues for payment. What works for you?"

Ms. Jones: "Well, I can pay for a part of this, but not all of it. Can we do this treatment a little bit at a time?"

Financial Coordinator: "No. That would not be in your best interest. Dr. Jameson is going to be providing eight veneers across the front teeth in the upper part of your mouth. You want to do these all at once so that the length and the color and the fit are just right. You are interested in getting a beautiful smile, and so are we. The veneers need to be done all at one time.

How much of an initial investment would you be able to make."

Ms. Jones: "Oh, I guess I could give you $2,000 at the start. But that would delete my savings and I'd have to pay out the rest."

Financial Coordinator: "OK. That would work. You can write us a check for $2,000 today and we can access a line of credit for you with our financing program. Then we can finance the other $2,000. Then, you would only be required to pay about $50 or $60 per month. Would that work for you?"

Ms. Jones: "Yes. It would."

Financial Coordinator: "Great. Let's complete the application right now."

THE FINANCING PROGRAM AS A VEHICLE

John is a great dentist. So are you. John's team is fabulous. So is yours. He goes to courses continually to upgrade his skill level. I'm sure you do the same. So, what makes the difference?

We think that one of the reasons he is able to provide so much quality restorative and cosmetic dentistry is that we can finance that dentistry through our healthcare financing program. Since cosmetic dentistry is not covered by dental insurance, for the most part, the patient must come up with the entire fee.

Offering the options that I addressed in chapter one, we make it possible for most anyone who wants and needs cosmetic dentistry to receive it. We don't have high level executives in our practice who want a new smile. We have "salt of the earth" people who want the best. They just need a way to pay for it—a way that fits into their particular financial situation.

I work with several plastic surgeons and many dentists who concentrate their practices in the area of cosmetic treatment. They want a patient to pay for the services up front. They tell me that if a patient owes them money, that somewhere down the road the person seems to find aspects about their cosmetic change that they do not like. Perhaps this is true. If a person owes you money, he/she may find and express fault with the treatment as an attempt to get out of paying the remaining balance. (This could be true with any treatment, wouldn't you agree?)

If a person owes you money or wants to have a balance excused, he/she will try to blame you *for something* so that you look like the bad guy and he/she looks like the good guy. A patient may—subconsciously—be embarrassed about poor money management. He/she may try to transfer a feeling of personal guilt to a feeling of blame to you.

SUMMARY

If you follow the recommended financial policy, no one will owe you money. No one will have an outstanding balance with you. Payment will be complete by the time the treatment is complete. If they owe money it will be to a separate entity, not you. This will lead to pleasant relationships, ones that are based on mutual benefit. You win—the patient wins. Stress is reduced for both parties. That is one more way to kindle or rekindle the joy of dentistry.

When Patients Complain About Your Fees

"Remind yourself that angry clients probably have a need that isn't being met and believe you have the ability at least to start the problem on the way to being solved."

— R O B E R T A C A V A
D I F F I C U L T P E O P L E

"**H**aven't your fees gone up, Doc?"

This *classic* statement by numerous patients whether or not you *have,* in fact, gone up on you fees can be upsetting. Many dentists and team persons are nervous about going up on fees because they don't want to face this question.

A careful analysis of fees needs to be done every six months. Why? To determine if any of your costs of operation and/or costs of a procedure have gone up. If your costs go up but your fees don't, profits are reduced. The one who usually gets a slash in salary is the dentist. Right!

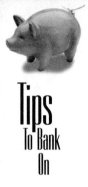

Tips
To Bank
On

Being over busy can
begin to squeeze patient
time, increase overhead,
and produce stress.

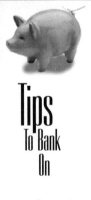

Tips
To Bank
On

. . . see fewer patients
in each day
doing more dentistry
per patient . . .

When you analyze your fees, you may find that they are just fine. However, if they need to be adjusted three, five, 10 percent or whatever, do so. Then know, as a team, that your fees are equitable and that they are *in line* for your area and that they reflect the quality of care you are offering.

When we first go into a practice to consult, and every time thereafter, we do a thorough analysis of the practice. We analyze each *system* and all of the statistical data. Before we go in—and during consult number one—the dentist and the team members begin setting goals for each of these systems.

Once we know where they are at the moment, and where they want to go, then we begin designing and teaching a plan of action to help them accomplish those goals.

Often, we see practices so busy that they can't even imagine putting in the necessary time to *clean up* their systems. They are seeing huge numbers of patients and have a hard time seeing people expediently. New patients have to be *put off* much too long; hygiene patients cannot be seen in a timely manner; major procedures are put off too far because the appointment book is stuffed full of smaller appointments—lots of them!

Being *over* busy can begin to squeeze patient time, increase overhead, and produce stress. The dentists and team members need to orchestrate a plan to increase revenue while decreasing both cost of operation and stress. Improving case presentation will lead to a higher acceptance of treatment recommendations and will continue to focus on high quality patient care. These in turn will lead to more comprehensive care, longer appointments, less stress for patient and provider.

Dentists must get out of the *habit* of thinking that high numbers of patients per day is the only way to be productive. It isn't. In order to spend more time with patients and on certain procedures, you may need to see fewer patients in each day doing more dentistry per patient and seeing those patients for fewer visits. But, remember—you do *not* want the profit margin of the practice to drop one percent.

Dr. Charles Blair, of Charlotte, N.C. has proven to me beyond a shadow of a doubt, that the single *best* way to increase practice profitability is to increase fees. If a practice is *full* of existing and new patients, increasing fees by 10% may cause a small percent of patients to go elsewhere. However, the practice would have to lose 20 to 25 percent of its patient family before bottom line profits would be negatively impacted. (according to Dr. Blair) If the practice increases fees by 10% across the board without adding other additional overhead items, the *bottom line* profits of the practice will increase over 25%. (for practices whose overhead is 60–65%)

I must tell you that I have recommended 10% increases in hundreds of practices but have *never* had 20 to 25% of the patient family leave—not if the practice focuses on quality throughout and has invested in great relationships with patients.

If you want to increase profitability by increasing your fees by 10%, you must be prepared for possible negative response by your patients. You must be strong—and ready—for a *few* people to leave your practice to go to a lower priced competitor. However, I have rarely seen this happen. Everyone on the team including the dentist must agree that seeing fewer patients in a day, doing more dentistry per patient, and seeing the patients for fewer visits is a desirable goal.

The verbal skills of how to deal with patient objections about fees are very important. You do not want people to leave you. You do not want people to be hostile about your fees. And so, how you handle the *very normal* complaints about fees will make all the difference in the world. Remember communication is the bottom line to your success with anything, including discussions about fees.

Example

> **Patient:** "Haven't you guys gone up on your fees since my last visit?"

> **Team Member:** "Yes, Ms. Jones, there has been a slight increase in our fees. Our costs of operation have gone up and, therefore, our fees have done the same. We refuse to compromise the quality of our care, and so, we carefully position our fees to reflect our commitment to the best".

> **Patient:** "Well, it seems like every time I come in here it costs more."

Team Member: "No, not every time. But I can appreciate what you are saying. When the cost of a procedure goes up, we increase our fee in order to cover those costs. We prefer to do this rather than use cheaper materials. Cheap materials produce average dentistry, and Ms. Jones the last thing in the world that we want to do is put average dentistry into you mouth."

INSURANCE AND FEES: USUAL AND CUSTOMARY

I don't think a dentist hates anything more than the classic letter from the insurance company telling his/her patients that a doctor's fees are above the usual and customary. Wow! It makes the dentist feel angry that a third party is coming between his/her relationship with a patient and it may make the dentist feel badly that the patient may have a misconception about the legitimacy of the presented fee.

One other issue can arise. If letters from the insurance companies are sent to the patients and if the patients call or make a scene in the office, the team members can become *gun shy* real fast! They begin to think, "Hey, maybe our fees *are* too high." or "Our poor patients can't pay for that treatment if the insurance company isn't going to pay, so maybe we should drop our fees."

That kind of mindset and attitude on the part of the dentist or the team members can lead to financial suicide.

The answer to complaints about fees is *not* to lower the fees. Upon reevaluation of your fees, your patient flow, your cost of operation, and your desired mode of operation, more than likely your fees are just fine or, they may still be a bit too low. For the most part, dental fees are equitable and fair.

The following steps need to be taken, however, so that you can deal professionally with the complaints that you are going to get.

1. The team needs to practice the verbal/communication skills of handling the patients' objections.

2. Create a letter that can be sent to patients when a protest about usual and customary occurs. (Fig. 8–1)

3. A letter needs to be placed into the practice armamentarium to send to insurance companies and to the state insurance commissioner to *protest* their intrusion into the patient/dentist relationship. (Fig. 8–2)

Usual and Customary Letter:

Dear Patient:

It has come to my attention that your insurance company has sent you a letter stating that my fees are "above usual and customary". I can understand how you would be confused and upset by this letter. Therefore, I am happy to provide a response to give you some information that may shed some light on this issue. I have sent a letter to your insurance company, a copy of which is enclosed for your review.

We appreciate dental insurance, and we believe that it is a wonderful supplement to a person's dental healthcare. However, it is not meant to be a *pay all,* only a supplement. As such, the amount paid for the premium determines the amount of available benefits. The more paid, the more received. The less paid, the less received.

Another point of confusion is about how an insurance company determines *usual and customary.* Their fees do not reflect any standard of care, but rather are a *median fee* based on fee schedules from all dentists in a designated area, which can include several different zip codes. This median fee, again, does not take into consideration an individual practitioner's own costs of operation or standard of care. Therefore, the fees are arbitrary and average rather than carefully determined.

We do our very best to provide above average care to you and to all of our patients. Our fees express an equitable exchange of value—fair fee for excellent services.

Sincerely,

Figure 8–1 Patient "usual and customary" letter

Insurance Company Name
Street
City, State Zip

Dear _____ :

I have recently been informed that your company has taken the liberty to inform a number of my patients, who are insured under your program, that you think that my fees are above the _usual and customary_ or _average_ rate for the community in which I practice.

I have verified my fees with the National Dental Advisory Service fee profile for this area and can verify that my fees have proved not to be in excess of those of my peers. I do believe that you are entitled to communicate to your policy holders. I further believe that you have an obligation to communicate the truth. Your company has determined in it's adjudication policies that it is unwilling or unable to pay for the quality and standard of dental care that the insured has chosen.

I would like to request, therefore, that you seriously consider re-phrasing your communication to accurately reflect your company's ability to reimburse. Otherwise, please cease and desist with your present communications which are inaccurate and intrusive in the dentist/patient relationship.

Sincerely,

John H. Jameson, DDS

cc: Insurance Commissioner, State of _____
       Patient

Figure 8–2 "usual and customary" letter for the insurance company and insurance commissioner

SUMMARY

There isn't a dentist in America (or anywhere in the world) who likes losing a patient. It kills you. I wouldn't want you to be any other way.

But, do *not* "let the minority rule the majority". Don't think that because one or a handful of patients protest about your fees that you are going to go *belly up*. Not raising your fees when *your* own costs of operation goes up *will* make you go *belly up*. And then, who wins? Not the patients, because you aren't in business anymore.

Put a mirror up to your practice. Are you epitomizing quality throughout? If not, make adjustments where necessary. Visualize the patient's experience with you and make sure each and every visit matches your idea of excellence. Then, set your fees accordingly.

Study communication skills so that you can present fees and overcome objections. Provide care to be proud of and let your fees stand as a clear indication of your practice of excellence.

Devising A Collection System for Past Due Accounts

"Realize the importance of getting the money in.
Do not be sentimental about this;
you are in business, you deserve to be paid
for the service you give, and you should be."

— PETER GLAZEBROOK
HAPPINESS AND FULFILLMENT IN DENTISTRY

If you follow the advice given in the preceding chapters, then you will "get out of the banking business". I am sure that you have realized that I would encourage you to remove yourself from carrying any accounts receivable except for a very short turnaround on insurance payments if you are taking assignment of benefits. No private pay accounts receivable. What a stress relief!

However, you may presently have some past due accounts or some accounts may "slip through the cracks" from time to time even though you have an excellent financial policy/system in

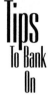

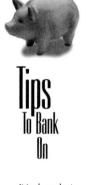

place. Therefore, a careful, sequential collection program for the recapturing of these accounts must be put into place and followed with persistence.

DEVELOP A COLLECTION SYSTEM THAT GETS RESULTS

Devise a foolproof system for discovering immediately when an account is overdue. Run an aged accounts receivable list each month and carefully evaluate each account to see the amount past due, the date of the last payment, and the amount of the last payment. Double check any formal financial arrangement to see if the patient is abiding by an agreed upon financial arrangement. (Fig. 9–2)

Establish a fair time schedule to determine the speed with which requests for payment should be made. Once you establish the time schedule, follow it with consistency. With a 30-day payment requirement a bill becomes past due on the 31st day. If bills/statements are sent monthly and a 30-day billing cycle is in place, 45–60 days may pass before payment is received. A 15-day cycle may need to be instituted.

When an account becomes delinquent, based on the decided length of time, a rebilling charge should be filed. However, notice of intent should be made in advance of such a charge. This notice can be a printed message on statements, stickers, or letters or notices and should always be acknowledged as a part of the system when original arrangements are made. It is always best to inform a patient of expectation before the fact.

Every evening, before the day is finished, the business administrator needs to review the patients who are coming into the practice the next day. She will identify any persons who either need to make a payment that day or who have a past due account that needs to be collected.

At the morning meeting or at the beginning of your day the business administrator makes sure that the appointment coordinator knows who will be paying that day and how much is required . In addition, she will identify those past due patients so that the he/she can be escorted into the business administrator's office for a private discussion of the past due account. Obviously, the goal is to get a written agreement on how the account will be settled.

Example Let's say that Ms. Patient owes $248 and that the account is 60 days past due. She is coming into the office today for an emergency appointment. The business administrator has identified the fact that Ms. Patient is coming at 10:00 A.M. and that she has this past due account of $248. When Ms. Patient arrives, the appointment coordinator or whoever is greeting the patient says the following to Ms. Patient,

"Ms. Patient, Jan, our business administrator has some paperwork that she needs for you to complete. We have a few minutes before the doctor sees you. Let me show you into Jan's office."

or

Before the patient leaves the office that day, make sure that she is escorted into the business office. The business administrator must have the chance to negotiate that settlement. The best way to collect an account is face to face.

In establishing a financial policy, firmness is essential. Offer the appropriate flexibility to meet the financial needs of your patients but be firm in adhering to that policy. Remember that firmness and fairness to both parties, consistency, and persistence are the keys to successful collections.

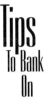

Tips To Bank On

The best way to collect an account is face to face.

A COLLECTION TIME LINE

Experts in the field of professional collection offer many helpful strategies to accomplish the greatest results in your collection efforts. They know how long and how hard you sometimes have to work to get an account collected. Therefore, they recommend a specific time line for successful collections to take place.

The following is the *best* time line as suggested by professional collection agencies. You are not a professional collection agency, but it would make sense to follow the guidelines of the people who do this for a living and who are only paid if they collect your account. They have to find ways to accomplish results or they are out of work.

Once again, let me stress the fact that the key to excellent collection of past due accounts is to follow a specific protocol. The following is the ideal collection time line.

At 31 Days Past Due

Collection procedure should begin at 31 days past due via telephone and/or letter. The thrust of this message should be simply that the account is past due and that payment is necessary.

At 45 Days Past Due

A second letter and/or telephone call needs to be sent or made. This message should be a request for payment within 15 days.

At 60 Days Past Due

A third letter and/or telephone call should be made. This message is a firmer one. The message is direct and states that payment is required and expected immediately.

At 75 Days Past Due

A fourth letter and /or telephone call is made—one that is firmer yet. This is an either/or confrontation; either the bill is paid or you will be forced to turn the account over for legal action.

At 90 Days Past Due

Three months of collection efforts have occurred—120 days have passed since the service has been rendered. A fifth letter is sent, no telephone call. This letter tells the debtor about the action that is *going* to be taken—legal action, collection agency, small claims court, etc. When the letter is sent saying that action *will* be taken—do so! Otherwise your efforts are wasted and your credibility is defused.

Management of an effective collection system takes careful planning as well as consistency and firmness in administration.

Tips To Bank On

Management of an effective collection system takes careful planning as well as consistency and firmness . . .

In addition, an understanding of people, an understanding of personality differences, and an understanding of the psychology of collecting is essential. The following criteria underlie successful collection.

- Be prompt and consistent.

- Increase firmness as the account delinquency increases.

- Have appropriate messages in letters or notices.

- Be aware of individual differences and needs.

- Have a knowledge of the legal requirements of collecting.

In creating collection letters or making collection calls, messages must be clear but courteous; firm but fair; positive rather than negative; persistent but not offensive; solid but not rigid.

MONITORING YOUR COLLECTION SYSTEM AND FINANCIAL ARRANGEMENTS

Establish a tickler file (Fig. 9–1) for your financial arrangements—January through December. After each financial arrangement is made, fill out a financial arrangement card. (Fig. 9–2). Place it in the appropriate place in the tickler file. This file will be assure the accurate tracking of each account. It will prove to be a very time-efficient method of monitoring your accounts due.

When you place a card in the tickler file, give the patient a five-day grace period before you make a telephone call about the past due account. In other words, if a payment is due on the 20th of the month, place a financial card in your tickler file on the 25th. Then, if a payment has not been received by the 25th, make your call. Review your tickler file every day. If a payment has been made, make note on the card of the date of the payment and the amount received.

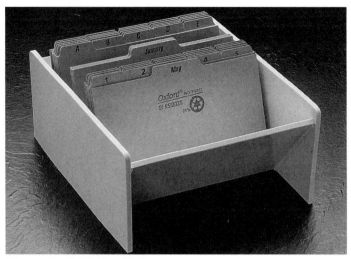

Figure 9–1 Tickler file

FINANCIAL ARRANGEMENTS CARD

Patient: _____ Date: _____
Guarantor: _____ Address: _____
Phone: (Home) _____ (Business) _____
Total: _____ Financial Agreement: _____
_____
_____
_____

Date Due	Amt. Due	Amt. Paid	Date Paid	Date Contacted	Comments

Figure 9–2 Financial Arrangement Card

If a payment is not received on the assigned day, (remember, you have given the patient a five-day grace period) call the patient and arrange a new due date. Record the new date on the financial card. File the card on the new date due. If you do not receive payment on the new date, make a second telephone call.

```
┌─────────────────────────────────────────────────────────────────┐
│ Guarantor's Name:_____        │
│ Phone: (home) _____ (business)_____         │
│ Total Balance:_____ Financial Arrangements:_____   │
│ _____ │
│ _____ │
├──────────────────────────────┬──────────────────────────────────┤
│ 1st Call:                    │ 2nd Call:                         │
│ Date: _____            │ Date:_____                  │
│ Payment Due:_____        │ Payment Due:_____             │
│ Date Due: _____          │ Date Due:_____                │
│ Last Payment Date:_____   │ Last Payment Date:_____        │
│ Amount Paid:_____         │ Amount Paid:_____              │
│ Notes:_____               │ Notes:_____                    │
│                              │                                   │
├──────────────────────────────┼──────────────────────────────────┤
│ 3rd Call:                    │ 4th Call:                         │
│ Date:_____             │ Date:_____                  │
│ Payment Due:_____        │ Payment Due:_____             │
│ Date Due:_____           │ Date Due:_____                │
│ Last Payment Date:_____   │ Last Payment Date:_____        │
│ Amount Paid:_____         │ Amount Paid:_____              │
│ Notes:_____               │ Notes:_____                    │
│                              │                                   │
└──────────────────────────────┴──────────────────────────────────┘
```

Figure 9–3 Call Form

Example: "Ms. Jones, this is Cathy with Dr. Jameson's dental office. Ms. Jones, during our conversation last Friday you indicated that you would be placing a check in the mail that day. We have no record of receiving that payment and I was concerned."

If the patient makes a partial payment, call them. Thank them for the payment that they did make. Then ask for the balance of the payment.

Payment Agreements

Date Due	Name	Telephone	Amount Due

Figure 9–4 Payment Agreement

Example: "Thank you, Ms. Jones, for your $50 payment. We appreciate this. However, our agreement was for $100 this month, and I was calling to see when we could expect the balance of your payment."

Let the person know that the agreement was for a different amount and that you need to get a commitment for the balance. This is critical because otherwise, the patient will think it is okay to send the smaller amount. Then your arrangement will stretch on forever.

Figures 9–2, 9–3, and 9–4 are examples of tracking devices that are workable. Choose one that works best for you—and use it consistently.

SUMMARY

Establish a protocol for collection and stick with it. The professional management of past-due accounts begins with excellent organization.

Collecting Past Due Accounts: Written Communication

*"The most important moment
in the life of a letter is not the moment it is written,
but the moment it is read."*

—NORMAN KING
PAST DUE: HOW TO COLLECT MONEY

Written communication with your patients who have a past due account is a very important step in receiving payments and in controlling your accounts receivable. It may be the only communication you will have with some accounts. In this chapter, I will give step-by-step instructions on how to administer the written part of collections. Written communication is used for the following purposes: (1) to notify the person of the overdue account and (2) to remind the person of the status of the account.

There are four phases of collection. Your written and your verbal contacts with your patients will follow and fit into these four phases:

- Notification of the past due account.

- Reminder of the past due account.

- Negotiation on how to settle the account.

- Action to be taken if compliance is not obtained.

THE NOTIFICATION PHASE

When an account becomes 31 days past due, the patient's statement needs to notify them of the delinquency. Be brief and to the point with your message. A stamped or computerized notice on the statement is appropriate. (Fig. 10–1)

PAST DUE

PLEASE SEND PAYMENT

BY RETURN MAIL

Figure 10–1

An alternative to the stamped notice on a statement would be a straight-forward handwritten message on the statement indicating the past due status. There's something pretty effective about the fact that you take the time to write a personal note on the statement. The patient will realize that you aren't just sending your statements off the computer without ever looking at them.

Use a bright color of ink for your handwritten note so that it will stand out when the patient reads the statement. (Fig. 10–2)

Dear Mr. Patient:

Your bill of $125 was due on July 6. Our records show that your account is now more than thirty days past due. We appreciate your attention to this matter and will look forward to receiving your payment by return mail.

Thank you,

Business Manager

Figure 10–2

Note: Each time during a collection letter series when you contact a patient, inform the patient of the amount due, the date the payment was due, and the length of time payment has been past due.

If you do not receive payment after this initial notification, move into the second phase of collection—*the reminder phase.* Fifteen days should be the time allowed between your first notification of the past due account and your second notice—*the initial reminder.*

THE REMINDER PHASE

The reminder phase of the collection process begins when notification has obtained no results. A series of notices and letters making a request for payment needs to be sent in a systematic manner.

During this *soft* phase of collection, your message should *assume* that the patient intends to pay but has simply overlooked the bill. This series of notices can include several types of correspondences: (1) Form letters (2) Stamped notices on statements (3) Pre-printed notices (4) Personal Letters.

The following are some examples of each.

Tips To Bank On

. . . your message should assume that the patient intends to pay but has simply overlooked the bill.

FORM LETTERS

A form letter is a non-personal way to *remind* the patient of the debt. This form can be a pre-printed, computerized, or a copied form. The patient owing you will see this as an impersonal, standardized process but may be stimulated to take action by the nudge. (Fig. 10–3)

Dear Mr. Patient:

Our records indicate that your account is past due. A balance of _____ is _____ days past due.

We would appreciate your attention to this matter.

Sincerely,

Business Manager

Figure 10–3

STAMPED NOTICES

Stamped notices on the statements can encourage action. These will have a stronger effect if they are in a different color— i.e., *red*. (Fig. 10–4 and Fig. 10–5)

PAST DUE

PLEASE SEND PAYMENT

BY RETURN MAIL

Figure 10–4

> # REMINDER:
>
> Your account is
>
> PAST DUE
>
> We look forward to
>
> receiving your check
>
> TODAY!

Figure 10–5

PRE-PRINTED NOTICE

Pre-printed stickers can be attached to the statement or pre-printed inserts can be produced that will deliver different messages. Use of several different bright colors of paper can bring attention to the notice. (Fig. 10–6)

> ## Your account is past due
>
> ### PLEASE REMIT!

Figure 10–6

Of the four types of notices, the personal letter is most widely used and is the most effective. *The other forms are to be used only once.* After that, they become ineffective.

However, the personal form letter can be a series of letters reminding a patient of the status of the account. These letters should become more urgent and stronger as the account ages. All personal reminder letters need to be courteous, but they do become more specific and more intense as time passes.

PERSONAL REMINDER LETTERS—
A SUGGESTED SERIES

The personal letter should be non-threatening, informal, and congenial. The following is an example of a series of personal letters that can be used to deal with a delinquent account. (Figures 10–7, 10–8, 10–9, 10–10, and 10–11)

Dear Mr. Patient:

In reviewing our records, we find that you have an outstanding balance of $248 for services provided on _____.

You may have overlooked your previous statement. Therefore, we wanted to bring the status of your account to your attention.

We would greatly appreciate your attention to this past due account and will look forward to receiving your check so that we can keep your record clear.

If your payment and this letter have crossed in the mail, please accept our thanks for your payment.

Sincerely,

Business Manager

Figure 10–7

Dear Mr. Patient:

Perhaps you have overlooked your bill for $248 for the services we provided for you on _____.

We would appreciate your attention to this past due account and will look forward to receiving your payment.

Thank you,

Business Manager

Figure 10–8

Dear Mr. Patient:

We have not heard from you regarding your $248 past due account. Perhaps you have overlooked or misplaced our previous notices. Therefore, because we are sure you want to take care of this account, we are sending this letter reminding you of your past due balance.

We appreciate your business and will appreciate your attention to this past due account. We look forward to receiving your payment in the next few days.

Thank you,

Business Manager

Figure 10–9

Dear Mr. Patient:

Your account of $248 is now 60 days past due. We have reminded you of the status of this account several times in the past two months.

Once again, we remind you that your account is past due and request your immediate attention to it.

If there is a problem—please know that we are here to help. Your telephone call will be appreciated.

Thank you,

Business Manager

Figure 10–10

Dear Mr. Patient:

We, again, call your attention to your now seriously past due account of $248. Your account is now _____ days delinquent.

Notices as well as detailed statements have been mailed to you several times.

We need to have this matter brought to a close. We will appreciate your payment.

Thank you,

Business Manager

Figure 10–11

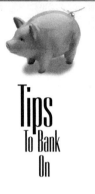

Tips To Bank On

Request that action be taken.

In this phase of the collection process, present the problem, the amount due, and the amount of time it has been past due. *Then request that action be taken.* This phase does not make any specific appeal. Compromise is not offered. Continue to assume in your correspondence that the patient intends to pay but has inadvertently overlooked the bill. You want to keep the patient on your side. You do not want to antagonize the patient. If the patient becomes irritated, the chances of being paid are reduced.

If notification and reminder do nothing to move a patient to action, then move your collection efforts to a stronger phase. Dr. Carl Caplan states in his *Encyclopedia of Dental Practice Management* that "the dental practice should not falter in its enforcement of a collection policy. It is not unfair to expect patients to meet their financial obligation. The dentist does not want to develop a *soft touch* reputation."

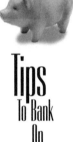

Tips To Bank On

You want to keep the patient on your side.

THE NEGOTIATION PHASE

No Payment? What do you do now? Negotiation for the settlement of the account can *and should* take place.

Your initial efforts to collect an account *assumed* that the patient *would* pay. You *just knew* that the statements had been misplaced or that there had been some confusion. You have tried to give the patient the *benefit of the doubt*. However, no payment has been received and no effort has been made to settle the account. In a stronger effort to settle the account, you need to find out the reason for the non-payment and negotiate a payment arrangement that is comfortable for the both of you.

You must move into a stronger mode of operation in your collection efforts. Each correspondence in this aspect of the collection sequence must be carefully planned and must be a part of an intensifying sequence of letters. Even though your efforts are getting firmer, you still want to *try* to maintain a good relationship with the patient. This will give you a better chance of settling the account. This is a tough balancing act—getting firmer while still maintaining a good relationship.

Your goal is to arrange a discussion with the patient regarding the resolution of the account. Each account must be treated individually. The purpose of this series of letters is to schedule a discussion appointment and come to terms with a payment agreement.

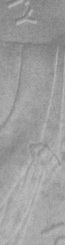

Tips To Bank On

Your goal is to arrange a discussion with the patient regarding the resolution of the account.

THE PSYCHOLOGY OF COLLECTION

In his book, *Past Due, How to Collect Money,* Norman King suggests that an understanding of the psychology of collection is critical to the success of such efforts. A variety of emotional appeals can be used during this portion of the process. Mr. King suggests that some common emotional appeals might be "sympathy, pride, justice, self-interest, cooperation/discussion, and fear."

SYMPATHY

Collection letters that appeal to the patient's sympathy try to make the patient aware of the fact that the dentist and the practice have provided a service both in treatment rendered and in the extension of credit. Now, because of the patient's inability or unwillingness to take care of the account, the practice is in a difficult position.

The effect of such an appeal letter is to draw on the person's *sympathy*. If this is a person with an *understanding heart*, this type of appeal will be effective for you.

Be cautious with this type of an appeal. If the appeal is not handled with expertise, the letter might appear *whiny* and the effect will be less than favorable. But, if your letter is carefully constructed and can petition a person's sincere interest in your situation, payment could result. (Fig. 10–12)

Dear Mr. Patient:

In order to maintain comfortable fees for our patients and in order to continue to provide the best possible dental care, we must constantly work at controlling our costs of operation When you send your payment for your outstanding balance of $248, we will no longer need to invest in statements, reminders, and postage. We will, then, be able to pass those savings on to you and to our other valued patients in the form of affordable, quality care.

Working with us on the resolution of your past due account will help all of us control the rising costs of healthcare.

We look forward to receiving your payment. Thank you for your cooperation.

Thank you,

Business Manager

Figure 10–12

PRIDE

Collection letters that appeal to a patient's sense of *pride* conjure a sense of guilt for having avoided or *pushed aside* a legitimate debt. The majority of your patients will have a sense of pride and a sense of responsibility about their debts. They will be—for the most part—men/women of their word.

Therein lies the power of the appeal to a person's pride. You have *assumed* that their integrity is in tact, and that circumstances have made it difficult to meet responsibilities. Most certainly, they do not *intend* to default on this balance.

Make note of how faithful with payment the patient has been in the past and how much you respect their attention to their account. The appeal to pride is effective with many people. (Fig. 10–13)

Dear Mr. Patient:

We have been so grateful for your continued loyalty and for your consistently prompt payments in the past. Please know that we have appreciated this.

Currently, we find that your balance of $248 is _____ days past due. We have made several attempts to inform you of the delinquency of this account. We value and respect you. Therefore, we are requesting an appointment to discuss a solution to bring the account to a current status. Please call our office today to schedule an appointment with me to negotiate a comfortable settlement of your account.

I will look forward to your call.

Thank you for your immediate attention to our request.

Business Manager

Figure 10–13

JUSTICE

Collection letters that appeal to a patient's sense of *justice* try to make the person owing the money feel that he/she is not treating the creditor justly by his/her action, or by a failure to act. The main impetus of such a letter is to emphasize that a valuable service has been rendered in a timely fashion and that you, as the creditor, believe and encourage *above board* business relationships. (Fig. 10–14)

Dear Mr. Patient:

In our recent letter to you, we asked for payment of your delinquent account in the amount of $248. We fully believed that we would receive the payment.

Knowing that you are a person of your word, we were surprised when the payment did not arrive on the date upon which we both agreed. As we discussed during our financial consultation, we do not carry long term accounts on our own books. By not abiding by our agreement, you have placed us in a very difficult position.

I am sure we can look forward to your attention to this past due account.

We would appreciate your prompt payment.

Business Manager

Figure 10–14

Tips To Bank On

"Sell an idea to the emotion and back it up with logic."

—TOM HOPKINS
OF SCOTTSDALE, AZ

SELF INTEREST

Collection letters that appeal to *self interest* have a strong impact on most people. This type of collection letter would be used best at the end of a collection letter sequence. It is a more intense letter than previous efforts.

The self interest letter combines an appeal to both the emotion and to the logic. Tom Hopkins of Scottsdale, AZ, whom I referred to earlier, believes that you have a stronger impact if you "sell an idea to the emotion and back it up with logic." Therefore, combine these two appeals in your *self interest* correspondence. The debtor must realize that it benefits him/her to take care of the account and that their credit standing might be damaged otherwise. At this point, do not be specific about the action you will take if the account is not rectified. (Fig. 10–15)

Dear Mr. Patient:

On several occasions, we have contacted you regarding your delinquent account of $248. We have not heard from you and are wondering why.

We placed trust in you by financing your dentistry in our own office. We are disappointed that this trust has not been upheld.

You are aware, I am sure, that mishandling of credit makes it difficult, if not impossible, to maintain those privileges in the future. In addition, poor credit ratings can negatively affect you for a long time to come.

We are sure that you will want to take care of your debt so that your good credit will be restored. This, of course, will benefit both of us. We want to reestablish that trust we once placed so confidently in you. Place your check in the mail today so that we can immediately resolve this issue.

We appreciate your prompt attention to this matter.

Business Manager

Figure 10–15

COOPERATION/DISCUSSION

What you are trying to obtain through your consistent, carefully planned collection effort is an opportunity to discuss the situation so that a resolution can be developed. You *want* to work this out! You are asking for cooperation from the patient and are willing to give the same.

Collection letters that appeal to or request a discussion come at the end of your collection letter series. It is, simply, an offer to sit down, one on one, with the patient to plan a settlement.

This type of an appeal is straight forward, mature, and will bring positive results in many cases. The letter simply opens the

Dear Mr. Patient:

Maintaining good oral health is critical to a family's overall health. We congratulate you for having realized that fact and for providing this care for yourself and for your family. Maintaining a good credit rating with our practice gives you the assurance that this type of care can continue.

You can certainly understand our position. In order to reestablish good credit with our practice, it will be necessary for you to honor the agreement we originally made. We have, on numerous occasions, sent you statements and reminders about the status of your account. These notices were very clear in their message that payment was due and payable on the date given.

May we ask that you mail us a check for the overdue amount? If, for any reason, this can not be provided, won't you, please, extend us the courtesy of phoning our office so that we can discuss a comfortable resolution?   Let's develop a plan of action that is a win/win for each of us.

We look forward to your call. We want to work with you.

(302) 321-4355.

Business Manager

Figure 10–16

door for the discussion. Arrangements for settlement will be made during the discussion. (Fig. 10–16)

Your previous letters of increasing intensity have led you to this point—the point where a discussion is encouraged. Once the discussion is arranged, plans for resolution of the account are made. You have moved out of the mode of notifying, reminding, appealing. Now you are ready to negotiate.

OPTIONS FOR SETTLEMENT

There are several options available for negotiation of delinquent accounts. Some of these options are as follows:

1. **Immediate Payment** This is the ideal solution. It indicates that the account will be paid in full—immediately. This is the ideal. But, at this point in the patient's payment history, the likelihood of this settlement is rare.

2. **Extended Payment** Be careful with this offer. Remember the length of time and the efforts you have already put forth to resolve the issue of the late payment. If the patient does not have an excellent explanation for the delinquency of the account or if proof of his/her willingness to pay cannot be presented, be wary of this offer. If you do make such an offer, extend the account for 30 days only.

3. **Postdated Checks** Postdated checks can be collected. This offer comes when the patient expects funding at a specific time. You must be able to establish if the expected income is real or imaginary. This is, of course, difficult if not impossible to do.

   The benefit of the postdated check is that you have the payment in hand. The downside of the postdated check is that should the postdated check bounce, you are back to your original problem. However, Bob Peterson, Director of Operations for Merchant Credit Adjusters of Omaha, Nebraska says that in his collection agency they encourage postdated checks because 98% of their postdated checks clear the bank. He says, "Get those postdated checks!" Mr. Peterson goes on to say that he starts all of his weekly staff meetings telling his collection professionals to get postdated checks on those accounts that they are trying to collect, because the results are so positive when they can get that check in hand.

"When you receive a postdated check, this creates a different relationship than does a *regular* check," says Peterson. "This does not represent that funds are currently available to cover the check. A postdated check changes a check from a demand instrument to a time instrument and the check is not payable until that specified date."

The Fair Debt Collection Practice Act, or Public law 95-109, September 20, 1977, Section 808 clearly states that credit grantors can ask for postdated checks. To check on the legality in your state, contact your state banking officials.

Peterson goes on to say, "A person who writes a postdated check is responsible for notifying the bank of the postdated check. The check is to be dated for the date when the transaction is to take place."

4. **Scheduled Payments** This is probably the most common method of settlement. With this option, a schedule of payments is established that will fit into the patient's monthly budget and will satisfy the practice. Ultimately, of course, a total resolution of the account results.

   Try to collect at least half of the balance immediately, then split the remaining balance over a couple of months.

5. **Consider Electronic Funds Transfer** during the negotiation phase of collection.

Example: A patient owes $800. You negotiate a series of payments whereby the patient pays $400 immediately and $200 on the fifteenth of the next two consecutive months.

Notice that an exact amount and an exact date have been established. This is critical. Write down the agreement on a financial agreement card (Fig. 9–2) and place in the tickler file. Keep a copy and give or send a copy to the patient. Then, if you have not received the scheduled payment, pick up the phone and make a call to the patient stating that you have not received the scheduled payment and are concerned.

The recording of this type of information and your conscientious follow-up are critical to the success of the agreement. Use that tickler file!

The following recommendations for tracking your collection efforts are made by Skylar Financial Control Corporation of San Francisco, CA:

1. Record all your collection conversations.

   a. Without a record, you cannot remember the status of an account when you call again.

   b. Your version of a conversation will be valid in court when you can show you regularly recorded conversations in writing.

2. Use the calendar or tickler file for any follow ups:

   a. If payment is promised on a certain date, mark your calendar or tickler file for that date and call if payment is not received.

   b. Similarly, note any action that is supposed to occur in the future, such as "patient is due to get a job in a month and start paying".

FEAR

You have appealed to a host of emotions. You have encouraged a person to respond to your notices, reminders, and efforts to *work with them* on the resolution of the delinquent account. Most people will have responded to one or the other of your appeals. Once discussion is initiated, collection procedures cease.

However, with about one person per hundred a willingness to pay does not occur. Some people really will not have the ability to pay. Others will refuse to pay or to honor their responsibility to you.

Up to now you have approached the person with an *assumption* that he/she is going to pay. Now, you must *assume* that they are not going to do so. You should still try to persuade the person to take care of the debt, but it is now appropriate that

179

you notify them that stronger measures *are* going to be pursued. This is your most intense appeal—the appeal to the sense of *fear.* It is a letter that demands action.

This letter is the final letter in your series of correspondences with the patient. It is, also, the first step in forceful action. In this letter, you let the person know that you are serious, and that you have taken this as far as you are going to take it within your own office.

THE DEMAND LETTER

Notice that this appeal to fear is firm, direct, and serious. However, the door is not completely closed for settlement outside of the law. (Fig. 10–17) This final appeal includes three specific steps:

1. A synopsis of previous efforts to collect

2. Your decision to turn the account over to professionals

3. A last opportunity to settle the account

Dear Mr. Patient:

Our records indicate that your balance of $248 is now 120 days past due. Our efforts to contact you and to negotiate a comfortable settlement of this account have produced no results.

Therefore, unless we receive a payment for the total amount of your delinquent balance within 10 days from the postmark of this letter, we will be forced to turn your account over for legal action.

Avoidance of this legal action is in your favor. We encourage you to contact our office immediately. Otherwise, we have no choice but to proceed with alternate measures.

Business Manager

Figure 10–17

SOME FURTHER GUIDELINES

Always control emotions when you are involved with collection procedures. Control your anger, your hostility, your resentment. There is a fine line between solid and acceptable collection procedures and defamation. Make sure that:

- All of your information is valid.

- Do not make derogatory remarks and do not accuse the patient.

- Do not use profanity. Do not profess anger.

- Address the letters specifically to the debtor, personally.

- Include an *out* in each letter.

SUMMARY

Collection is tough! It is not *usually* one of the *favorite* responsibilities in a dental practice. However, (1) if you have a firm financial policy in place; (2) if financial arrangements are carefully made and written down; (3) if you have a collection system in place that can be followed with success, the efforts will be more palatable and more successful. Remember: The key to success in collection is persistence and consistency.

The key to success in collection is persistence and consistency.

The Telephone:
Its Role In Effective
Collections

*"The telephone is, in many instances,
the most effective form of account collection."*

—Dr. Charles Blair
Marketing for the Dental Practice

If the guidelines in the initial chapters of this book are followed, you will have very few, if any, accounts receivable and very few past due accounts. But, when you begin to "change your financial life", you will probably have some past due accounts that will need your attention.

Getting a very solid handle on who owes the practice, how much they owe, the length of time that the account is past due, and the date of the last payment is essential information for good collection to take place. Discussing the account with the patient face to face is the best way to collect those past dues. The next best way is through excellent collection telephone calls. The least effective way is through the written communication. A

Tips To Bank On

The goal of your collection calls should be to maintain a good relationship with your patients while letting them know that you expect payment from them.

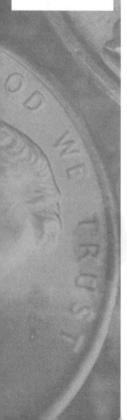

combination of all three is usually necessary to reach the people and to establish the mode of payment that will work best for that particular person.

It is not always possible to converse with a patient face-to-face, and so making collection telephone calls is critical. The manner in which you handle those calls and the verbal skills used make the difference.

The goal of your collection calls should be to maintain a good relationship with your patients while letting them know that you expect payment from them. You want to keep lines of communication open, and you want to get to a point where negotiation of an acceptable settlement is reached. Ultimately, both the team member and the patient should feel good about the call and the resulting negotiation. The end result of an effective collection system is accounts receivable control.

WHEN MAKING COLLECTION TELEPHONE CALLS, REMEMBER:

1. Identify yourself.

2. Immediately state the purpose of your call.

3. Make a statement about the status of the outstanding account (amount past due, days past due, and the date of last payment)

4. Ask questions to discover the problem.

5. Review the original payment arrangement.

6. Use active listening to determine objections.

7. Work out or negotiate a settlement for the problem.

8. Summarize the agreement. Record the conversation and the agreement.

9. Thank the person for his/her cooperation.

10. Keep a copy of the agreement for your record and mail the patient a copy.

11. Keep your records updated each time you correspond with the debtor.

12. Follow up on any action you have said you would take.

13. Stay calm. Losing your temper, becoming angry, or getting defensive will only cause the debtor to do the same thing.

14. Stay in control of the conversation by asking questions and by keeping the person involved in the conversation.

15. When you ask a question, stop and let the person make a response. Don't feel like you have to fill voids in the conversation. Pausing at appropriate times keeps you in control.

16. Speak slowly, calmly, and clearly.

17. Make sure that a firm agreement has been reached before the conversation ends.

18. Make sure that you keep an accurate record of all transactions and all conversations, then follow up on any agreements. Do what you say you will do.

19. Maintain a positive attitude. It's okay to expect patients/debtors to abide by their agreements. You respect them. You can expect respect in return.

20. Persevere!

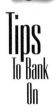

Tips To Bank On

Make sure that a firm agreement has been reached before the conversation ends.

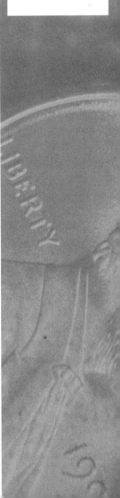

COLLECTION TELEPHONE SCRIPTS

Here are some guidelines that will help you get ready for the challenge of making telephone collection calls. The better you are prepared, the greater your success. The greater your success, the stronger your confidence.

1. Pre-plan your call. Be completely prepared. Have all necessary data in front of you. Have the chart in front of you. Get your financial agreement form or card so

that you will know what was—or was not—agreed upon. On this card will be the results of past collection efforts so that you will know exactly what has been done, what was said, and the results of previous conversations.

2. Review the patient's history—clinical and financial—before you pick up the telephone. If you need to have a discussion with people in the clinical or business area who have dealt with this person or this situation, do so in advance of the telephone call. Your success and your confidence will be in direct proportion to your preparedness. Don't get *hung out there* because you were not prepared and did not know the appropriate information.

3. Be sure not to put the patient on the defensive. Great communication skills will be vital. You must be an excellent listener. You must know the strategies of negotiation. You do not want the person to become defensive because, if they do become defensive, they will become angry. They will not be as interested in working out an agreement with you. In addition, you risk losing the patient and having him/her *bad mouth* you all over the town.

    (I know! You are saying, "Well, if this person owes me money and if he/she gets rough, I don't want them in my practice anyway!" I know. However, we are going to approach this collection thing in a positive way with the goal of a quality negotiation of settlement and of a continued relationship with the patient.)

4. Focus the conversation on taking care of the patient. Let the person know that you are interested in him/her and that you want to work out an arrangement that is as good for him/her as it is for you.

Key principles in a negotiation process are as follows:

1. Discover what the person's needs are at this time.

2. Listen as they share their concerns and their needs. Listen without judgment.

3. Define your own needs—what you are and are not willing and able to do.

4. Make it clear that you are interested in making this arrangement beneficial to the patient. (People need to know, "what's in this for me.")

5. Do not settle for an agreement that is not good for both parties. A win/win resolution is a must.

Sample Script for Collection Calls:

"Hello, Ms. Jones? This is _____ from Dr. _____'s office. Ms. Jones, in reviewing our records, we find that your balance of $_____ is _____ days past due. We have not received a payment since _____. Is there a problem?"

Listen to her answer. Repeat back to the person what you think you have heard him/her say. Express a sincere concern for the problem. Empathize, but do not sympathize. Understand the situation but don't feel sorry and back off from expecting payment.

"So, you have had some unexpected expenses that have made it difficult to fulfill your responsibility to our office, is that correct? I understand how that sort of thing can happen, and I am sorry you have had these difficulties. However, our agreement called for a payment of $_____ due on the _____. In order for our accountant to maintain his records, I must be able to tell him when we can expect your payment of $_____."

If the patient becomes angry or defensive, stay calm. Don't get upset. Don't hang up. Do everything possible to make sure the conversation stays on an even keel. Make sure you end the conversation in a positive, peaceful, settled manner.

If the patient becomes defensive, or if the patient does not show an inclination to be cooperative, use an "I" message to express your problem. An "I" message expresses your problem in terms of how it is affecting you in a negative way. It is not a *put down* message that places the person on the defensive. You also want the patient to know that you are interested in creating a situation where both of you benefit.

> "Ms. Jones, I felt concerned when we did not receive the payment you agreed to make to our practice, because late payments mean late penalties for you. This will add to the total amount due, which I am sure you would like to avoid. Therefore, let's work together to come to an arrangement that is comfortable for both of us."

Always thank the person for their agreement. Repeat the agreement to make sure that you have a common understanding of that agreement. Inform the patient that you are recording the agreement and that you will be sending them a copy of that agreement.

> "Thank you, Ms. Jones, for you cooperation. Let me review our agreement to make sure we both have the same understanding. We can expect to receive a payment of $83 on the 15th of January, on the 15th of February and on the 15th of March. The March payment will clear your account with us. Is that your understanding? Are you comfortable with that agreement? I will make a note of this for our files and I will send you a copy of this agreement."

Make sure to record the information, make a copy and send it to the patient. Include a self addressed envelope for the payment. Place a note in your *tickler* file so that you will be alerted as to when you are to expect that patient's payment.

During Telephone Collection Calls

While the telephone has proven to be very effective for collection, it must be used carefully and professionally. Be cognizant of the Telephone Harassment Laws and abide by those regulations. Violation of the regulations can lead to loss of telephone service, fines, and/or criminal action.

The following need to be avoided:

1. Calls, anonymous or otherwise, made in a frightening, abusive, or harassing manner.

2. Calls that interfere with the use of the telephone by other customers.

3. Calls for purposes that are against the law.

4. Calling at unreasonable hours of the day or night. (Do not call before 8 A.M. or after 9 P.M.)

5. Making one call after another to the same person.

6. Calls to people other than the debtor to discuss the past due account.

7. Calls that make threats.

8. Calls making false accusations about damaging a person's credit rating.

9. Calls stating that legal action is going to take place if, in fact, it is not.

10. Calls demanding payments for a debt that is not actually owed.

11. Calls that give inaccurate information about the original agreement.

Summary

Your efforts to collect via the telephone *will* be effective. Practice the skills outlined in this chapter. Gain confidence as a result of your study and practice.

Written communication is vital, but not as effective as face-to-face or telephone communcation. This is a significant part of effective collection—the telephone.

When All Else Fails!

"There are many countless ways of attaining greatness, but any road to reaching one's maximum potential must be built on a bedrock of respect for the individual, a complete commitment to excellence, and a total rejection of mediocrity."

—BUCK RODGERS,
FORMER VP OF MARKETING FOR IBM
GETTING THE BEST

You have pursued a past due account with persistence and consistency. Nothing happens! No response! No payment! Now what?

You, as the creditor must now choose between three stronger efforts to collect your money: (1) small claims court, (2) a collection agency, or (3) an attorney.

Let's analyze these three methods of collection. What are they? How do they work? When is each of these processes appropriate? What can you expect?

SMALL CLAIMS COURT

Small claims court is a vehicle for the small business owner—the dental professional—to use when (1) an account is past due, (2) efforts to collect privately have failed, and (3) the amount owed is under $1000. (Check with your state for this maximum amount. It differs from state to state.)

Small claims court is used *only* when all of your own pursuits have been ignored. With small claims court you need not hire an attorney. You may appear in court yourself or a designated member of your team may appear to represent the practice. There are fees for this service, but they are much less than attorney fees.

The court appearance will take time out of work. However if there are enough accounts, or if there is a high enough past due amount, the time spent could prove to be very cost effective. Many debtors are encouraged to pay when they realize that you are serious about the matter.

In most states, small claims court will handle cases of less than $1000. However, there is some variance among states, so you will need to check your area to see the limitations. In some states, cases can be pursued only if the disputed amount is above $1000. In other states, there is no such thing as *small claims court* but rather *magistrates court*. In addition, certain states will not allow a team member to appear in court for the dentist if he/she is incorporated. In that case, the dentist or an officer of the corportion would be required to appear.

Call your local authorities at your city hall to find out which court will handle cases of your type and spend a bit of time investigating the protocols of your particular state. Being prepared will save you time and money in the long run.

One of the benefits of this type of court is that the time spent in court is minimal. The actual presentation of the case takes but a few minutes. A supervisory judge will either rule on the case himself or will assign the case to an attorney or an arbitrator. Most of the cases today are decided by an arbitrator. This person in most instances will make a decision based on the specific instance and will apply fairness and objectivity.

In most states, the creditor (the dentist) would file the suit. In other words, you or your practice can do this without the assistance of any third party. In fact, many states will not allow a third party, such as a collection agency, to file suit in small claims court. Again, check into your state regulations.

A statute of limitations is enforced in most states—usually four years. Hopefully, you would have filed suit long before the four-year statute of limitations. Why?

1. The sooner you begin and the more persistent you are with your collection efforts, the better your results will be.

2. Judges in small claims court are more likely to rule in your favor if you prove that you have made careful, consistent efforts to collect. Showing that you are *on top* of your business will be to your advantage.

3. If the debtor *goes under* you will be more likely to receive at least *some* payment if you are one of the first to file a suit.

HOW DOES SMALL CLAIMS COURT WORK?

There are five steps to take to participate in small claims court. They are as follows:

1. Pay a fee to file the suit.

2. File your statement.

3. Serve the debtor with papers.

4. Present your records of proof.

5. Arrange a date for the hearing.

Pay a Fee to File the Suit. There will be nominal fee required for this entire process to go forward. The fee will range from $5.00–$15.00. There may be some other fees that you will be responsible to pay. These fees can be added to the amount owed by the debtor.

File Your Statement. Each court system will require different types of paperwork. The dentist, who is now the creditor will become the *plaintiff,* in legal terms. The dentist (or the office) will fill out a statement which will give information, such as your name, the debtor's name, the past due amount, the date you provided the services, and the history of your collection efforts.

Your statement will be handed to the court clerk who will type the statement. This will then become the *claim of the plaintiff.* You will sign one copy of this statement, one copy will be given to the judge, and one copy will be given to the debtor, who will now become the *defendant.*

The claim of the plaintiff is served to the defendant. If this person cannot be found, he/she must be sought through more extensive methods, such as tracking services provided by individuals or certified or registered mail.

The *tracking services* are provided by people such as a sheriff, a marshal, or another law enforcement person. This would be a person who has no involvement with the case in any way. The fee for this service is usually under $25.00. The papers must be served to the defendant in person. The papers cannot be left with another person or in the mailbox. If the server does find the person or makes an effort to give this person the papers, but the debtor refuses to take them, then the server puts the papers down and leaves. Obviously, stronger methods are not appropriate.

Certified or registered mail can be used in most states as a method to serve the defendant with papers. The court clerk usually does this. The defendant must sign for the mailed papers. If this person is *accustomed* to collection methods he/she may not sign for the document. It will be up to you to contact the court clerk to find out if the defendant has received the papers. You must do this before your day in court.

You set your court date when you file your statement. You need to leave enough time between your filing and the court date for the defendant to have been served. It is not always necessary but it is wise to have all of your records of service and of collection efforts with you when you appear in court. Gather this information and be able to present it in an organized fashion.

Small claims court is not as highly structured nor is it as highly intense as *regular* court. The fact that the debtor has been brought to court over this past due account makes him/her more likely to pay. You, the defendant, and the arbitrator may all sit down together to discuss the issue. No one else will be involved. If the debtor, or defendant, does not *show up* for this day in court, what happens?

If this happens, then you will be awarded a *default judgment.* You think, "Well, I'm back to square one." Actually, you are better off because you have the power of the court behind you. You have a judge's decision and because this debt is now on record, you can do things that you couldn't do before.

COLLECTING PAYMENT
ONCE A JUDGMENT IS ACQUIRED

Once you receive a judgment, there are several ways in which the money can be collected from the defendant:

- Wages

- Bank account

- Automobiles and other vehicles

- Property (except residence)

Before wages or other property can be accessed, or levied, you must have a court order. This is called a *writ of execution.* You receive this writ from the court clerk following the passing of the judgment. You will then send this writ to the sheriff or marshal or another law enforcement person in the debtor's county. You will pay a fee to this law person and you will give him instruction as to where the debtor or the property can be found and what he is supposed to seize or collect.

To levy on a bank account you will need the following: (1) the original and one copy of the writ of execution and (2) a letter of instruction about what to do: "levy this person's bank account", or "levy this person's wages", etc.

If the debtor has no job or no bank account, then levying vehicles or property is the next option. Obviously, this is difficult and takes a great deal more time and effort.

If you are going to pursue a levy on a person's wages, here are a few things to note. This is known as a *garnishment*. The act of levying wages is called *garnisheeing* them. The employer is known as the *garnishee*. Limits may apply as to how much money can be withdrawn from each paycheck. Most states do not allow an employer to dismiss an employee because of garnishment.

The employer, although an innocent third party, does become the legal trustee or custodian of the debt owed by his employee. The court action is a restraint on him, not allowing him to pay full wages to the employee but rather transferring a part of the moneys to the said creditor.

In many states, once a writ of execution is obtained for levying of wages, the court orders the garnishee (debtor's employer) to appear in court to discuss the issue of the owed monies. This does not usually go over very well with the employer, as you might imagine. If he/she fails or refuses to appear in court then the court pursues the garnishee—or the employer—a formerly innocent bystander! This is an acceptable and workable method of collection, but use it as a last resort.

Levying a person's bank account or personal property is called *attachment*. Limits are usually set as to how much can be attached. Attachment is a legal provision that allows the creditor to access a person's banked funds or available properties. The purpose of this legal action—the attachment—is to prevent people who do have available funds and/or properties from ignoring their responsibilities and spending their money on themselves or on other things besides the debt.

The requirements for attachment vary from area to area, but most states do make this collection apparatus available. The process of acquiring an attachment is similar to garnishment. All procedures flow through the court itself, once a judgment is received.

Why would you consider attachment?

- The debtor is *hiding* in an effort to avoid the creditor or legal action.

- The debtor has left your state to avoid legal action.

- The debtor makes an effort to remove or sell property to avoid legal acquisition of those properties.

Benefits of Small Claims Court

The advantages of small claims court are that the process is quick and simple. There are costs involved, but those costs are much less significant than either a collection agency or an attorney. With the power of the court behind you, much greater leverage is in your favor. With this leverage, you can do just about as much as a collection agency or an attorney.

Tips On Small Claims Court

- Allow for at least two weeks for your court date.

- Be on time for your case—even if you have to wait once you get there.

- Be able to spend time in court, if need be.

- Be prepared. Bring all your documents with you to court.

- Be concise. Give a precise, accurate, short description of your information.

- Don't become angry. Don't lose your cool.

- Do not slander your defendant.

A COLLECTION AGENCY

Sometimes you do not want or need to pursue an account in small claims court. The amount of the debt may be too small to offset the *cost* of your lost office time. If this is the case, you might consider the employment of a collection agency. This, of course, would occur only after you have done everything you could possibly do to collect the account through your own efforts.

Once you make the decision to turn an account over to the agency, you are *out of it*. You should stay out of the way and should not do anything else to try to collect the account. This action—turning the account over for collection—will probably end your relationship with the patient. But, at this point, you have probably decided to do this anyway. Do everything you can to settle the account, but if your efforts fail and you turn the account over to a collection agency, step out of the way and let them do their work. By his/her actions, the patient has chosen this action.

You may find that the professional collector has a stronger effect on the debtor, and that they can get more done. In other words, because there is no personal relationship between the collector and the debtor, more pressure can be applied which will result in positive action.

Many of the same steps of collection that you have used will be followed by the professional collector; telephone calls, a sequence of specific letters, and so on. However, the pressure placed by the professional will be taken more seriously, in most cases.

WHICH AGENCY

How do you decide which agency to employ? There are over 5000 collection agencies across the country. Make sure that the agency you choose has an office in the location of the debtor. Check references and make sure that the agency has a good reputation. You do not want to employ an agency that has developed a reputation of improper handling of debtors. In other words, the agency must be professional—not overly aggressive.

Be sure that the agency does not misrepresent itself with words such as "United States", "Federal", "National", etc. The agency you choose should operate a *free demand* service. This would indicate that the creditor—the dentist—would prepare a triplicate form, one for the debtor, one for the agency, and one for the practice. This form states that if payment isn't received, that the collection agency will take any and all necessary steps to collect the money.

A set amount of time is given—usually 10 days—and the form would state that if payment isn't received within that 10 days that action will be taken. If, by some chance, you receive payment within that 10-day period of time, you must let the agency know so that action is not taken. Thus, it is called *free demand service.* You would pay nothing to the collection agency if the patient pays within the assigned time frame.

If, however, you feel that the debtor will not settle the account within 10 days, the account should be placed as a *regular collection service,* and action will begin immediately. The fees charged by collection agencies vary from state to state and from agency to agency. Be absolutely sure that you check out the fee schedule before you turn any account over to an agency. Their fee schedule should be provided at your initial contact with them. Ask for it.

If the agency must access the skills of an attorney to complete a collection transaction, the fees—obviously—will go up. If this action must be taken, you will be informed of the action, as well as the additional fee.

YOU NEED TO KNOW

The collection agency, after they have spent some time pursuing an account, may recommend that you accept a partial settlement. This is, always, your decision. If this recommendation is made to you, bear in mind that the debtor wins out. He/she hasn't paid you anything. Now, you are being asked to settle for less than the owed amount. In addition to the reduction in debt, you will be paying a fee to the collection agency.

Example: Say a person owes you $1000. The debtor agrees to pay 50% or $500. In addition to this lowered amount, let's say that you are paying 30% to the collection agency. You will be paying $150 to them for their services. Thus, on the $1000 amount you are owed, you would receive $350. The debtor wins. But, in some cases, this is better than nothing at all and having at least pursued the account through a professional means you gain some satisfaction as to the *principle of the matter.* This person should not receive services in your practice from that point forward.

The negative information about this person's collection status will be placed on his/her credit record and will inhibit future loans for a period of time—usually seven years.

THE ATTORNEY

If you have pursued an account through all of the methods outlined previously, and if you choose not to access the services of a professional collector, an attorney can be hired to handle the legal pursuit of an account. The attorney will take such legal action as (1) litigation, (2) attachment, (3) garnishment, and (4) lien.

You, as the creditor, have the right to go to court to force a debtor to settle a past due account. When you work through an attorney, you usually can exert more pressure than if you were to handle this by yourself.

Just like you, the attorney goes through a specific series of letters—collection type letters. If the attorney receives no response from the debtor, then stronger measures are taken. The attorney notifies the debtor that he/she is going to take them to court. If no action is taken at that point, then court it is!

It will be expensive for you to have an attorney take one of your debtors to court. You need to discuss those fees and costs before the fact.

Gather your documentation—the clinical records, all records of collection efforts, information about the debtor—including information about the debtor's property, bank accounts, employment, income, etc. For you to be able to attach or to garnish you must know if the debtor owns property valued at least in the amount of the debt plus the expenses of the suit. You can usually gather this information from the attorney or the collection agency. This will help you make a decision about your actions. If there is not enough said property, then it really does not pay to pursue the account through the courts.

The use of an attorney and the court system is complicated. There are three specific stages of pursuit: (1) pleading the case, (2) trying the case, and (3) executing the settlement of the account.

In the first stage, the pleading of the case, the creditor—or the dentist—is represented by the attorney. The dentist becomes the plaintiff. All information is gathered, a petition is filed, and a summons is issued. The debtor can file an answer to this summons and set up his/her own defense. If there is no response or answer to the summons, a default judgment results.

In the second stage, trying the case, the trial takes place. Information is shared and a judgment is ruled. If the judge rules in favor of the plaintiff, the court determines how much is to be paid. In some states, an automatic lien on property is established.

In the third stage, the execution of the settlement, the court instructs a law enforcement person to collect the amount—often from the person's property. This property is seized and is put up for sale by public auction. The proceeds from the auction are turned over to the court, court fees are withdrawn, and the creditor receives the balance. If no property is available, the judgment is *docketed* for the future when property is available.

As was pointed out earlier, if the amount due is less than $1000 you are better off to go through the small claims court. There is less time and money involved and less headache.

The fees for the services of an attorney are high. Most attorneys will not work on your smaller debts. However, on those larger debts, this is a very acceptable method of collection.

As was discussed earlier, attachment and garnishment can result from the attorney's efforts.

BANKRUPTCY

You receive a Bankruptcy notice on one of your patients. Now what? Bankruptcy used to be a bad word. Now, it's commonplace. For the debtor, bankruptcy is the final chapter in trying to *spell relief* from indebtedness. It is a voluntary or an involuntary move on the part of the debtor to declare insolvency to the courts. When bankruptcy is declared, the creditors *line up* to divide assets, sell properties, receive pro rata percentages of payment relative to the size of each claim.

You *might* get a portion of *your* balance from the sale of the debtors assets. But, if you do receive any payment at all, it will probably be only a portion of the overdue amount. Historically, 10–15% receipt of the claim is the norm.

For the person declaring bankruptcy, getting out of debt and getting a fresh start are the advantages. Even the best business person may be caught in an unsolvable situation that makes it impossible to satisfy debts. Bankruptcy allows this person the opportunity to continue working to pay off debts. In addition, this gives the creditor some *hope* of payment or solution.

TYPES OF BANKRUPTCY

There are two main types of bankruptcy voluntary and involuntary. With the voluntary type, the debtor requests to be declared bankrupt. With the involuntary type, the person is forced to declare bankruptcy by creditors.

Business bankruptcy falls into two main types. They are Chapter X and Chapter XI. If a company is forced into bankruptcy by creditors, Chapter X is declared. If the company declares bankruptcy on its own, this is Chapter XI. Chapter X and XI involve businesses, not individuals.

Key Points About Chapter X

1. Chapter X is a forced bankruptcy.

2. Quick action is taken.

3. Liquidation of the business takes place.

4. All assets are sold.

5. Proceeds from the sale of assets are used to service debts.

6. Court costs, attorney fees, trustee fees come off the top.

7. The remaining dollars are spread among the declared debtors, secured and unsecured.

8. Secured means that the money owed is backed up with collateral—goods and or services (Banks have secured debts.)

9. Unsecured means money is owed, but there is no collateral. (At this point, there may be little or nothing left!)

10. An unsecured creditor can hope to receive 10–15% of the debt.

Key Points About Chapter XI

1. The firm requests the right to stay in business so that income can be generated to service debts.

2. The firm remains in business under the supervision of a court-appointed trustee.

3. After an in-depth study, the trustee decides whether or not the company should stay in business.

4. A plan of reorganization is made.

5. Once approved, the plan goes into action and debts are serviced as revenues are generated.

6. All *new* debts are serviced first.

7. Original creditors are not paid off until all new creditors are serviced.

8. The trustee approves all new purchases.

9. Old debts may not be paid in full.

10. If the company still fails, the courts will declare Chapter X.

So! What do you do when a patient declares bankruptcy?

1. If you have turned an account over to a collection agency and you receive a bankruptcy notice, contact your agency promptly and withdraw your claim. Otherwise, if the collection agency files the claim, it will receive a percentage of what *little bit* is recovered. Thus, you would receive a minuscule portion of your debt.

2. After you withdraw your claim from the collection agency, you must file your own claim with the bankruptcy court. You will fill out a *proof of claim* (provided by the court). Once completed, send it back to the court.

3. Then wait. The court will notify you as to the status of your claim. Hopefully checks will be sent to you as the assets are sold. Some time may pass, even years!

PERSONAL BANKRUPTCY

Two other types of bankruptcy do not deal with businesses but rather with individuals—Chapter VII and Chapter XIII.

The Bankruptcy Reform Act of 1978 has made it pretty easy for an individual to declare personal bankruptcy. Once bankruptcy has been declared and court proceedings begin, all creditors must *back off* and wait for results to be determined. A $60 fee is filed to declare bankruptcy. Since the Reform Act multitudes of personal bankruptcies have been declared.

Key Points About Chapter VII

Chapter VII bankruptcy is the voluntary declaration of bankruptcy by an individual. The person, the debtor, files bankruptcy with the court. The court then reviews the situation and decides *yes* or *no* on the declaration. If the court says *yes,* it begins the process of selling the debtor's assets and distributing the proceeds of the sale to creditors. Chapter VII allows the debtor to retain enough assets to *live—some* home equity, car, and personal items. Under this type of personal bankruptcy, the debtor cannot refile for bankruptcy again for six years.

Key Points About Chapter XIII

Chapter XIII bankruptcy involves people whose "principal income is derived from wages, salaries, or commissions". When the debtor declares himself insolvent and unable to service debts, bankruptcy is declared. This petition by the debtor, states that the debtor wishes to resolve all debts by reorganization, consolidation, or extension of those debts. This will be done out of future earnings.

The following steps are taken following the declaration of Chapter XIII bankruptcy:

1. A list of assets and liabilities is determined.

2. A *referee* is acquired and his/her fee is established.

3. The case goes before a judge or the referee.

4. All creditors meet. (10 days notice of the meeting is given)

5. The debtor is examined.

6. Witnesses testify.

7. A plan of action is determined.

8. The plan is accepted or rejected.

9. If accepted, the debtor continues to work to service debts.

10. Some payment adjustment may be made as to amount owed and amount actually paid.

11. The amount owed is paid to the court who then makes equitable distribution.

This type of bankruptcy is better than most. The rate of payment is higher than most bankruptcies. In some reports, indications say that 92% of debts will be serviced.

FOR THE CREDITOR

Without question, the Bankruptcy Reform Act of 1978 has made it easier to declare and *get by with* not servicing debts. For you, the dentist, the creditor—the act has made it more difficult to access receipt of debt.

We all know that if pushed too hard a debtor will *simply* declare bankruptcy and walk away from indebtedness or at least, put off payment of debts for long periods of time.

Ultimately, pursuing debts in the early stages and doing this consistently and effectively as outlined—is the *best* way to collect the monies owed to you for services rendered.

SUMMARY

You have made a financial arrangement. You have provided the service. You deserve to receive payment for treatment rendered. Being too timid about your collection procedures is *not* the answer.

It is not *your* fault if a person has financial difficulties, but it is your responsibility to pursue the account. Remember, the sooner you begin your tracking of and pursing of a past due account, the better chance you have of collecting it.

Review *all* steps of collections as previously outlined. Put these steps into an *action* plan that will work for you. Be firm, yet fair; Be tough, yet equitable; Be persistent! Be prepared! These principles are the key to successful collections.

Tips To Bank On

Be firm, yet fair;

Be tough, yet equitable;

Be persistent!

Be prepared!

Getting the Most Out of Your Collection System

"Focused action beats intellectual brilliance every time in the marketplace of human affairs."

— MARK SANBORN

We agree that collecting what you produce makes good sense. Having the revenues from completed dentistry sit on your books losing value is stressful as well as costly. Therefore, having a collection system in place that works, and works well, is good business and makes for happier dentists and happier dental teams.

Let's review some of the *musts* attached to setting up and maintaining an effective collection system. Here are *20 critical factors* that will let you get the most out of your collection system:

1. Have a written financial policy that everyone in the practice knows and understands. Make sure that your policy is good for the patients and good for the practice.

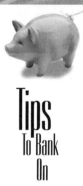

Tips
To Bank
On

Having the revenues from completed dentistry sit on your books losing value is stressful as well as costly.

2. Offer payment options that will meet the needs of the vast majority of your patients. However, make sure that you are not setting up a banking business within your practice. Offer options that will make the financing of your dentistry comfortable for your patients, and will not put you in a position of loaning money.

   You can't afford to loan money and run a financing business in your practice. In addition, you are dental professionals not banking professionals.

3. Get involved and promote a healthcare financing program. Make it easy for people to pay you. Have solutions available for *most* people's financial situations.

   These financial programs let the practice receive its money up front while letting patients have a chance to spread small monthly payments out over a long period of time. Thus, the patients will not be financially stressed by having to come up with large sums of money at one time.

   For most people, the decision to go ahead with the dentistry does not come down to "How much is the total investment?" Rather, saying yes to treatment often depends on "How much do I have to pay per month?"

4. Maximize your healthcare financing program by using the six strategies as outlined in chapter three. From your initial contact with a patient let them know your commitment to quality dental care and to convenient financing. Let your patients know that you do not want the financing of the dentistry to get in the way of them receiving the very best care possible.

5. Make financial arrangements with all patients prior to service. Prepare a written financial agreement that outlines not only the services to be rendered, but also the financial responsibility and the method of payment chosen. Then and only then will the person in the business office know how much to collect at each appointment. In addition, she will know the method of payment selected so that she can be prepared for the collection sequence at each appointment.

With careful and precise financial agreements written and placed carefully in the patient's record, the business administrator will be able to collect professionally and will not be scrambling at the last minute to ask questions of the clinical team, such as , "What did you do today? How much did you charge? How is the patient going to pay? What are you going to do next time? How much is that going to be? How will they pay." She will, also, never have to say to the patient, "Would you like to pay today?" or "How much would you like to pay today?" or "Oh, don't worry about that today. I'll send you a statement."

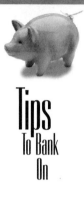

Tips To Bank On

Putting your head in the sand in relation to your past due accounts is poor business and does nothing to accomplish the goal of collecting what you produce.

6. Maintain an accounts receivable balance of no more than one to one and one-half times your average monthly production. This balance will be insurance balances for the most part. Do not let your past due accounts get out of hand. Run aged accounts receivable reports every month—separating your reports into 30, 60, 90, 120 days past due. Be aware of each account and the status of that account at all times.

   Dentists and business administrators need to stay in touch with one another about these accounts. Putting your head in the sand in relation to your past due accounts is poor business and does nothing to accomplish the goal of collecting what you produce.

7. Set a goal to have a 30-day turnaround of insurance claims. If you are computerized and are using electronic claims, your turnaround on money will be less than that. If you have insurance claims that are outstanding more than 30 days, you need to look closely at your insurance *system.*

   Approximately 50% of the revenue of the average dental office comes in the form of an insurance check. Therefore, as difficult as it may be to manage insurance, this crucial system within your practice deserves special attention.

   Make sure your *system* of filing and tracking insurance claims is without flaw. File each claim daily and make sure that if a claim becomes 30 days past due that you are in contact with the insurance company exploring the problem.

If you are not doing electronic processing of claims, do so, immediately.

8. Send statements every month to all people who have a balance with the practice—even people whose balance reflects an insurance balance.

When you are making a financial arrangement with a patient, let each one know that you will be filing the insurance as a service—but that if for any reason insurance has not paid within 30 days, he/she will be receiving a statement. Tell the patients that you want them to know the status of their account at all times.

From the beginning, let people know that you file insurance as a service to them. Let them know that they are responsible for their balances. If you wait to send statements after all insurance has paid—and if the person has a balance—too much time may have passed and the patient may be less than motivated to pay you. Keep them accurately informed as to the status of their account.

9. Place messages on your statements to notify the patient of the past due status, but do not kid yourself and think that this will be enough. A telephone call made at the 31-day past due point will accomplish much better results. The quicker you contact a person regarding the past due status of an account, the better your chances of collecting. Collection experts will tell you that the longer an account goes unattended, the weaker your chances of getting paid.

10. Using the letters included in this book, establish a clear, consistent sequence of collection letters. Remember to increase the intensity of the letters according to the past due status of the account.

These letters must be sent out like clockwork in order to access good results. The letters are not offensive. They are professional letters that follow the four stages of collection that must be adhered to if you are, indeed, going to collect those delinquent accounts. Remember those four

Tips
To Bank On

Collection experts will tell you that the longer an account goes unattended, the weaker your chances of getting paid.

phases: (1) Notification Phase, (2) Reminder Phase, (3) Negotiation Phase, and (4) If All Else Fails Phase.

11. Itemize your statements.

12. Collect the private pay portion of a patient's fee at the time of the service. Do not wait to collect the patient's portion after insurance has paid. This is financial suicide. Depending on how long you are waiting for insurance, you risk not being at the top of a patient's priority list of "Who's going to get paid this month?" Don't put yourself into this potentially detrimental situation.

13. If there is a balance after insurance has paid, send a statement the day the insurance check is received. Better yet, have a pre-authorization form from one of the bank cards or from your healthcare financing program. (Fig. 13–1) This pre-authorization will allow you to charge an insurance balance the day it presents itself.

14. Make it easy for the patients to pay you. On your statements, let people know that they can pay with a bank card. If your computer will not let you program your statements to say this, get a stamp. Also, VISA has stickers for statements that make it possible to pay in this manner. Or, produce inserts for your statements. (Fig. 13–2)

15. Place a due date on all statements. (Notice on your own bills at home that there is always a due date.) You will expedite payment by placing a due date on your statements. The due date should be within 15 days of the billing date.

16. At the end of every month divide the amount of money collected by the amount of dollars produced. This will give you the collection percentage for the month. Keep a running tabulation of this throughout the year. Maintain at least a 98% collection ratio. Set the goal—98% collection (or more!).

17. Have a person on the team responsible for accounts receivable control. Make sure that this person is analyzing your accounts receivable every month—all accounts.

Tips To Bank On

Set the goal—

98% collection!

You may modify you own billing statements to include the bank card payment authorization section of this sample billing statement.

Billing Statement

ABCD Medical Center
P.O. Box 12345
Anytown, U.S. 99999

John Sample Patient
1234 Any Street
Anytown, U.S. 99999

PATIENT NAME ______

ACCOUNT NUMBER ______

DISCHARGE/SERVICE DATE ______

BILLING DATE ______

PAYMENT DUE DATE	PAYMENT AMOUNT DUE	ENTER AMOUNT PAID HERE

BANK CARD PAYMENT AUTHORIZATION	
☐ ☐	Card Account Number ______ Expiration Date ______ Cardholder Signature ______

For your convenience, you may also pay by phone by calling 999-999-999

RETURN THIS PORTION WITH YOUR PAYMENT

DETACH HERE

DATE OF SERVICE	DESCRIPTION OF SERVICE	AMOUNT

BILLING DATE	PATIENT NAME	ACCOUNT NUMBER	PAYMENT DUE
Payments received after this date will appear on your next statement.	For questions concerning your outstanding balance, please telephone our business office M-F, 9:00 a.m.–4:00 p.m. at 999-999-9999.		

Figure 13–1 Example of statement to make payment on Bank Card (Credit: Visa)

Have a specifically outlined system of collection letters and collection telephone calls so that time does not pass without a patient hearing from you. If an account becomes 31 days past due, it is just that, past due. Begin your collection efforts right then.

18. Access training in the area of collection. Do not assume that just because someone is good in business

For Your Convenience We Accept VISA, MASTERCARD, DISCOVER, AMERICAN EXPRESS, AND HEALTHCARE FINANCING PROGRAM

Please Fill Out The Following:

☐ VISA   ☐ MASTERCARD   ☐ DISCOVER
☐ HCFP   ☐ AMERICAN EXPRESS

AMOUNT _____

CARD NUMBER _____

EXPIRATION DATE _____/_____/_____

SIGNATURE _____

Figure 13–2 Statement Inserts

administration that they will automatically be good at collection. There are specific skills that go along with the making and administering of financial arrangements. There are, certainly, specific skills related to the collection of past due accounts.

Let the talented person on your team who is responsible for this very important and very intricate system in your practice have the necessary armamentarium to carry out those responsibilities successfully.

Access books—such as this one, tapes, courses, and special consultation in the financial area of practice management. The dollars that you invest in your financial coordinator, in your financial system, and in your practice will come back to you multi-fold.

19. The person in charge of accounts receivable control needs specific time to make collection calls—time that is without interruption or distraction. These calls are not easy and need special attention. She will get more done in less time if she can earmark a certain number of hours—non-patient hours—for accounts receivable control.

This critical part of the practice must have attention. It's hard to pay the bills if the dollars aren't in the bank. But it

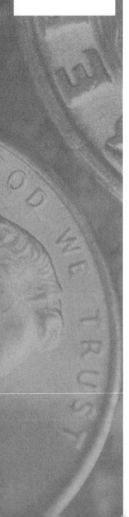

is hard to collect those dollars if the time is not scheduled for working on the accounts. Time well invested? I would say so!

20. Approach collection efforts with a positive attitude—a productive attitude. Know that it is OK to collect what you produce. Know that you have provided a service. There was an agreement for payment of the service. You are, simply, asking people to maintain their part of the agreement. If you expect to get paid, you will be. You never know what you will get unless you ask.

SUMMARY

Know that the very best way to collect an account is face-to-face. The second best way to collect an account is over the telephone. The least effective way to collect an account is by letter. All of these methods are a part of an effective collection system, but face to face is best. Therefore, getting and maintaining an excellent collection system within the practice is essential. Collect at the time of the service. Preventive management will save time and money in the long run.

And, Finally

*"Change is the law of life.
And those who look to the past and present
are certain to miss the future."*

—JOHN F. KENNEDY

Congratulations for purchasing this book and for getting to this, the last chapter. By doing so you are, obviously, interested in improving the business systems in your practice. You are aware of—but not afraid of—the financial challenges that face both you and your patients. Implementing the skills and strategies outlined in this book will help you to deal with these challenges in a positive and beneficial way.

Know that your practice is a conglomeration of systems—20 systems. Each of those systems must be carefully and caringly developed. Then, all members of the team must be committed to administering the systems consistently. Even though there are times when you must *flex*, do not let flexing become the norm.

If you do so, your systems will weaken and will fall apart. If one of the 20 systems is not working well, that will have a negative effect on all of the other systems.

For example, if you are not collecting what you are producing, you cannot continue to improve the clinical efficiency in your practice, because you will not be able to afford new and better equipment and instrumentation. If you are not collecting what you are producing, you cannot afford to hire and pay qualified employees so that your team is strengthened. And so on.

You have been given a path for developing a financial system in your practice. A good, workable financial policy was suggested. Healthcare financing programs were explained and you were encouraged to get involved with these programs. I suggested six ways to build your practice using a healthcare financing program and verbal skills, lots of them, were outlined for the presentation of these programs.

If you are interested in developing the cosmetic aspect of your practice, a brief review of the financing of cosmetic dentistry was suggested. This led to a discussion of how to overcome and handle the objection of cost—including some suggestions of how to handle your patient's complaints about your fees.

Devising a collection system in your practice is critical for the reduction of accounts receivable and for the continued *cleanliness* of your collection system. You may need to spend some time cleaning up old accounts, but once you do, you will never have to be in the accounts receivable business again, if you follow the instructions within this book.

The area of financing and collection need not be a dreaded/ feared/ ignored part of the management of your practice. You are providing a fabulous service to your patients. You are a healthcare business, and, as such, must run your business astutely. Getting and keeping control of your collection system is good for you and for your patients.

Remember, if you do not run a profitable business, you cannot afford to stay in business. Then, everyone loses, you and the patients alike. They need you and the services you are

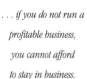

Tips To Bank On

. . . if you do not run a profitable business, you cannot afford to stay in business.

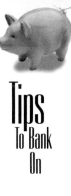

offering. *Collect What You Produce!* That makes it possible for you to continue to serve, and it makes dentistry much more fun.

Finally, stress will be controlled for all parties if the strategies of this book are implemented and followed. Stress can be controlled in the dental environment through excellent management and excellent communication.

I believe in you. Believe in yourself. Be the best you can possibly be—*now and forever.*

Call me!

—Cathy

Tips To Bank On

. . . stress will

be controlled . . .

Healthcare Financing Programs

Dent-A-Med, Inc.
1-800-262-3368
P.O. Box 1567
Fayetteville, AR 72702

Henry Schein Financial
   Services
(Med Cash)
135 Duryea Road
Melville, NY 11747
1-800-443-2756

CARECREDIT
1-800-300-3046 ext. 339
   Attn.: Derek
901 E. Cerritos
Anaheim, CA 92805

VISA
1-800-VISA-311

Norwest Financial
(Consult Your Local Directory
   For Listing)

American General Finance
(Consult Your Local Directory
   For Listing)

PulseCard, Inc.
913-345-2522
913-345-8456 (Fax)
9401 Indian Creek Parkway,
   Suite 470
Overland Park, KS 66210-2007

Health Group Services, Inc.
Transitions
Derek Hill, CA
BCE Place 181 Bay Street,
  Ste. 3500
P.O. Box 827
Toronto, Ontario M5J 2T3
CANADA
416-777-6069 (Office)
416-594-2514 (Fax)

Healthcare Creditline
P. O. Box 340038
Tampa, FL 33694
or
4014 Gunn Hwy.
Tampa, FL 33624
1-800-489-3279

Trend Systems
108 Brookes Path
Aledo, TX 76008
1-800-801-6419
1-800-795-7645 (Fax)

Paul Woody, E.A.
General Business Services
3205 NW 63rd Street
Oklahoma City, OK 73116
405-840-1751
Tax and Financial Consulting

Bibliography

Blair, Dr. W. Charles and John K. McGill, J.D. *The Blair/McGill Advisory*. Charlotte, NC. Blair, McGill & Company.

Caplan, Dr. Carl Michael. *Dental Practice Management Encyclopedia*. Tulsa, OK. PennWell Publishing, 1985.

Center, Dr. T. Warren. *Dentistry Today*. Montclair, NJ. Dentistry Today, Inc., 1990.

Gordon, Dr. Thomas. *Leader Effectiveness Training: The No-Lose Way to Release the Productive Potential of People*. New York, NY. Bantam Books, Inc., 1977.

Gordon, Dr. Thomas and W. Sterling Edwards, M.D. *Making The Patient Your Partner: Communication Skills for Doctors and Other Caregivers*. Westport, CT. Auburn House, 1995.

Hopkins, Tom. *The Official Guide To Success*. Scottsdale, AZ. Tom Hopkins International, Inc., 1982.

Jameson, Cathy. *Great Communication = Great Production.* Tulsa, OK. PennWell Publishing, 1994.

Jameson, Cathy. *Dental Practice Success Newsletter.* Ardmore, OK. Sprekelmeyer Printers, Volume 2, Number 1.

Jameson, Cathy and W. Paul Woody. *How To Work With General Dentists.* Oklahoma City, OK. General Business Services. 1996

Kelsay, J.D., Ed. *Collecting Medical Accounts.*

King, Norman. *Past Due: How To Collect Money.* Facts On File, Inc., 1983

McCormack, Mark H. *What They Don't Teach You at Harvard Business School.* New York, NY. Bantam Books, Inc., 1984.

Murphy, Kevin J. *Effective Listening: Hearing What People Say and Making it Work for You.* New York, NY. Bantam Books, Inc., 1987.

Oakes, Dr. Woody. *The Profitable Dentist.* New Albany, IN. Excellence In Dentistry.

Peterson, Bob and Bonnie. *Dental Practice Success Newsletter.* Ardmore, OK. Sprekelmeyer Printers, Volume 2, Number 2.

Visa. *Tools For Patient Payment.* San Francisco, CA. Visa U.S.A., Inc. 1995.

Woolery, Ph.D., Michael F. *Creative Communicators.* Glendora, CA. Royal Publishing, Inc. 1990.

Index

A

Acceptance, 105–106

Account status, 163–181

Accounting reduction for payment, 7

Accounts receivable administration, 29–32, 49–57, 209, 211, 213–214: account analysis, 49, 211; account transfer, 49–57

Accounts receivable analysis, 49, 211

Accounts receivable transfer, 49–57: telephone campaign, 52, 54; tracking devices, 52, 55

Accounts receivable, 29–32, 49–57, 209, 211, 213–214

Action to be taken, 156, 164, 180–181, 211: legal, 211

Active listening, 103–105, 123, 126–127

Added value (services), 120

Administration, 4–5, 29–32, 49–57: financing program, 4–5; accounts receivable, 29–32, 49–57

Agency selection (collection), 198–199

Aging accounts, 154–157

Answering objections, 122–125

Application for financing program, 51

Appointment payment, 7–8

Assignment of insurance, 8–9, 69

D

E

F

JAMESON MANAGEMENT GROUP

THE COMPANY'S MISSION AND VISION

The mission of Jameson Management Group is to serve the health-care industry as a consulting and lecturing service that provides both business and personnel management. The following is a statement of mission and purpose for Cathy Jameson and Associates and Jameson Management Group Consulting Services:

1. To make a positive difference in the lives of the professionals whom we have the privilege to serve.

2. To teach practice management with a heart.

3. To teach practical skills of business and personnel management.

4. To facilitate excellent relationships between and among team members—via the teaching of effective communication skills.

5. To help team members understand these communication skills and be able to serve patients better because of productive communication.

6. To integrate business systems that will lead the way to productivity and profitability for the practitioners and the entire team.

7. To teach systems that are time efficient, cost efficient, and will control stress.

Cathy Jameson provides in-office consulting services and seminars through her company, Jameson Management Group, Inc., located in Oklahoma. For more information, please call (405) 369-2501 or (405) 369-5555. Correspondence and inquiries can be sent to:

Jameson Management Group, Inc.
P.O. Box 488
Davis, OK 73030-0488